W0111686

CBS Confident Pharmacy Series

Pharmacognosy

Third Edition

for First Year Diploma in Pharmacy

(0807) Strictly Based on Syllabus as per ER1991

Question–Answer Type Notes and Board Question Papers (1996 to 2017)

Salient Features

❑ Total Confidence and 100 percent Success in Every Examination.

❑ Repeatedly Asked Board Questions Indicated in Brackets.

❑ Chapterwise Collection of Very Important Questions.

❑ Written in Very Simple and Lucid Language.

❑ Board Question Papers 2015–2017 given at the End of Text.

CBS Confident Pharmacy Series

Pharmacognosy

Third Edition

for First Year Diploma in Pharmacy

(**0807**) Strictly Based on Syllabus as per ER1991

V.N. Raje M Pharm

Principal
Gourishankar Education Society's
GES College of Pharmacy (D Pharm)
Limb, Satara, Maharashtra

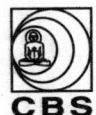

CBS

CBS Publishers & Distributors Pvt Ltd

New Delhi • Bengaluru • Chennai • Kochi • Kolkata • Mumbai
Hyderabad • Jharkhand • Nagpur • Patna • Pune • Uttarakhand

Pharmacognosy

Third Edition

ISBN: 978-93-86478-51-1

Copyright © Author and Publisher

Third Edition: 2018
Reprint: 2018, 2019, 2020, 2021
First Edition: 2010
Reprint: 2011
Second Edition: 2015
Reprint: 2016

Published by Satish Kumar Jain and produced by Varun Jain for

CBS Publishers & Distributors Pvt Ltd

4819/XI Prahlad Street, 24 Ansari Road, Daryaganj, New Delhi 110 002, India.
Ph: 011-23289259, 23266861, 23266867   Website: www.cbspd.com
Fax: 011-23243014   e-mail: delhi@cbspd.com; cbspubs@airtelmail.in.
Corporate Office: 204 FIE, Industrial Area, Patparganj, Delhi 110 092
Ph: 011-4934 4934   Fax: 011-4934 4935   e-mail: publishing@cbspd.com;
publicity@cbspd.com

Branches

- **Bengaluru:** Seema House 2975, 17th Cross, K.R. Road,
  Banasankari 2nd Stage, Bengaluru 560 070, Karnataka
  Ph: +91-80-26771678/79   Fax: +91-80-26771680   e-mail: bangalore@cbspd.com
- **Chennai:** 7, Subbaraya Street, Shenoy Nagar, Chennai 600 030, Tamil Nadu
  Ph: +91-44-26680620, 26681266   Fax: +91-44-42032115   e-mail: chennai@cbspd.com
- **Kochi:** 42/1325, 1326 Power House Road, Opp. KSEB, Kochi 682018, Kerala
  Ph: +91-484-4059061-65   Fax: +91-484-4059065   e-mail: kochi@cbspd.com
- **Kolkata:** 6/B, Ground Floor, Rameswar Shaw Road, Kolkata-700 014, West Bengal
  Ph: +91-33-22891126, 22891127, 22891128   e-mail: kolkata@cbspd.com
- **Mumbai:** 83-C, Dr E Moses Road, Worli, Mumbai-400018, Maharashtra
  Ph: +91-22-24902340/41   Fax: +91-22-24902342   e-mail: mumbai@cbspd.com

Representatives

- **Hyderabad** 0-9885175004 • **Jharkhand** 0-9811541605 • **Nagpur** 0-9421945513
- **Patna** 0-9334159340 • **Pune** 0-9623451994 • **Uttarakhand** 0-9716462459

Printed at Mudrak, Noida, UP, India

to

my beloved family

Preface to the Third Edition

The third edition of the now popular and successful book includes Board Question Papers 1996 to 2017. The book has been written to meet the requirements of students of Diploma in Pharmacy (D Pharm) in accordance with the new revised syllabus ER1991 prescribed by Pharmacy Council of India.

This book is small and humble effort has been put in for compiling necessary information on the subject. An attempt has been made to demystify and simplify the basic concepts for the students of pharmacy and to enable them get an evergreen success in MSBTE examinations.

The salient features of the present book are:

- Lucid and easy language
- To the point answers,
- Remembering facts in the simplest way, and
- Infusing confidence in the reader to appear in the Board Examinations.

Hence the series is named

CBS Confident Pharmacy Series

I am confident that this book will be useful to both the students and the teachers of Diploma in Pharmacy as well as the candidates desiring to succeed in competitive examinations for better job opportunities in pharmacy profession such as hospital pharmacists in PHCs, civil hospitals, etc.

Raje Vijay N

Acknowledgements

I express my heartfelt thanks to Prof Madan Jagtap, Chairman, Gourishankar Education Society, Satara Maharashtra, for consistent encouragement and inspiration for writing this book.

I wish to acknowledge the prompt and efficient help given by Prof Milind Jagtap, Mr Jaywant Salunkhe, Mr Appa Rajage, Mr Nitin Mudalgikar, and Mr Shrirang Katekar of Gourishankar Education Society, Satara.

I am also thankful to Shri Satish Kumar Jain, Chairman and Managing Director, and Shri RN Mandal, General Manager, Pune Branch, CBS Publishers & Distributors Pvt Ltd, for their sustained efforts and keen interest in the publication of this book.

I wish all my beloved students to have a great success in the Board Examinations.

Raje Vijay N

Syllabus

(As per ER 1991)

Pharmacognosy

1. Definition, history and scope of pharmacognosy including indigenous system of medicine.
2. Various systems of classification of drugs of natural origin.
3. Adulteration and drug evaluation: Significance of Pharmacopoeial standards.
4. Brief outline of occurrence distribution, outline of isolation, identification tests, therapeutic effects and pharmaceutical applications of alkaloids, terpenoids, glycosides, volatile oils, tannins and resins.
5. Occurrence, distribution, organoleptic evaluation, chemical constituents, including tests wherever applicable and therapeutic efficiency of following categories of drugs.

   a. Laxatives—Aloes, rhubarb, castor oil, ispaghula, **senna**.
   b. Cardiotonics—**Digitalis**, arjuna.
   c. Carminatives and gastrointestinal regulators—Umbelliferous fruits: coriander, fennel, ajowan, cardamom, ginger, black-pepper, asafoetida, nutmeg, cinnamon, clove.
   d. Astringents—Catechu.
   e. Drugs acting on nervous system—Hyoscyamus, belladonna, datura, aconite, ashwagandha, ephedra, **opium**, cannabis, nux vomica.
   f. Antihypertensives - Rauwolfia
   g. Antitussives - Vasaka, tolu balsam, tulsi
   h. Antirheumatics - Guggul, colchicum
   i. Antitumour - Vinca
   j. Antileprotics - Chaulmoogra oil
   k. Antidiabetics - Pterocarpus, gymnema
   l. Diuretics - Gokhru, punernava
   m. Antidysenterics - Ipecacunha

n. Antiseptics and disinfectants - Benzoin, myrrh, neem, curcuma

o. Antimalarials - Cinchona

p. Oxytocics - **Ergot**

q. Vitamins - *Shark liver* oil, amala

r. Enzymes - Papaya, diastase, yeast

s. Perfumes and flavouring agent—Pepermint oil, lemon oil, orange oil, lemon grass oil, sandalwood.

t. Pharmaceuticals aids—*Honey*, arachis oil, starch, *kaolin*, pectin, olive oil, *lanolin, beeswax,* acacia, tragacanth, sodium alginate, agar, guar gum, *gelatin.*

u. Miscellaneous—Liquorice, garlic, picrorhiza, dioscorea, linseed, shatavari, shankhpushpi, pyrethrum, tobacco.

6. Collection and preparation of crude drugs for the market as exemplified by **Ergot, Opium, Rauwolfia, Digitalis, Senna.**

7. Study of source, preparation and identification of fibres used in sutures and surgical dressings—Cotton, *silk wool* and regenerated fibres.

8. Gross anatomical studies of—Senna, datura, cinnamon, cinchona fennels, clove, ginger, nux vomica and ipecacuanha.

Contents

CHAPTER 1

History and Scope of Pharmacognosy

1. **Pharmacognosy (S. 98, 99, 01, 02, 03, 07; W. 97, 99, 00, 07, 08):** Pharmacognosy is defined as a systematic and scientific study structural, physical, chemical and biological characters of crude drugs including the study of their history, cultivation, collection and preparation for market.

2. **Laxatives/purgatives:** The drugs which promote defaecation are called laxatives, e.g. castor oil, senna, rhubarb, aloes, ispaghula.

3. **Cardiotonics:** The drugs which increases the force of cardiac muscles and stimulates the activity of heart are called cardiotonics, e.g. digitalis, arjuna.

4. **Carminatives (W. 05):** The drugs which expels the gases from GIT by increasing peristalsis are called as carminatives, e.g. fennel, coriander, cardamom, ginger, clove, cinnamon, clove.

5. **Astringents:** The drugs which cause precipitation of superficial proteins are called as astringents, e.g. black catechu, pale catechu.

6. **Analeptics:** The drugs which stimulates the central nervous system are known as analeptics or CNS stimulants, e.g. nux vomica, lobeline.

7. **Antihypertensives:** The drugs which reduces elevated blood pressure to the normal level are called as antihypertensive, e.g. rauwolfia.

8. **Antitussives:** The drugs which are used in the treatment of cough are called as antitussives/anticough agents, e.g. vasaka, tulsi, tolu balsam.

9. **Antirheumatics:** The drugs which are used in the treatment of rheumatism are called as antirheumatics, e.g. guggul, colchicum.

10. **Antitumour/anticancer agents:** The drugs which are used in the treatment of cancer are called as anticancer agents/drugs, e.g. vinca.

11. **Antileprotics:** The drugs which are used in the treatment of leprosy are called as antileprotic drugs, e.g. chaulmoogra oil.

12. **Antidiabetics/hypoglycemic agents:** The drugs which are used in the treatment of diabetes mellitus are known as antidiabetic drugs, e.g. gymnema, pterocaprus.

13. **Diuretics:** The drugs which increases the formation and excretion of urine are called as diuretics, e.g. gokharu, punarnava.

14. **Antispetics:** The drugs which kills the microbes when applied to living tissues are called as antiseptics, e.g. benzoin, nim, myrrh, curcuma, turmeric.

15. **Disinfectants:** The drugs which kills the bacteria and their spore when applied to nonliving tissue are called disinfectants, e.g. benzoin, myrrh, nim, curcuma, turmeric.

16. **Antimalarials:** The drugs which are used in the treatment of malaria are called as antimalarial agents, e.g. cinchona.

17. **Oxytocics/Echbolics:** The drugs which stimulates the uterine contraction and expel the contents of uterus are called as oxytocics, e.g. ergot.

18. **Vitamin:** Vitamins are organic substances present in small amounts in natural food stuffs and are essential for growth of body and normal metabolism, e.g. shark liver oil (vitamin A) amla (vitamin C).

19. **Enzymes:** Enzymes are the protein substances which catalyse various biochemical reactions, e.g. papain, diastase, yeast.

20. **Perfumes:** These are the substances made from natural or synthetic materials are used for creating a pleasant odour, e.g. rose, jasmine, sandalwood, citronella.

21. **Flavouring agents:** These are the agents used to give a pleasant flavour to the formulation, e.g. peppermint oil, lemon oil, orange oil, lemon grass oil.

22. **Pharmaceutical aids:** The substances which are of little or no therapeutic value but are essentially used in the manufacture of or compounding of various pharmaceutical products are known as pharmaceutical aids, e.g. honey, starch, acacia, gelatin.

23. **Crude drug (S. 05, 06, 08; W. 03, 05, 06):** It means the drugs occurring in natural forms.

24. **Source of crude drug:** Crude drugs are obtained from plant, animals or minerals which are known as source of crude drugs.

25. **Organised drugs:** The drugs which have a definite cellular structures are called as organised drugs, e.g. fennel, cinchona.

26. **Unorganised drugs:** The drugs which do not show a definite cellular structure are called as unorganised drugs, e.g. acacia, tragacanth.

27. **Aphrodisiac:** The agents which stimulates the sexual desire are called as aphrodisiacs.

28. **Technical products:** The drugs from natural source which are used in the industries like food industries are called as technical products, e.g. ginger, cardamom, caraway.

29. **Technical use:** The use of drug other than pharmacological use is called technical use.

30. **Substitute:** Substitutes are the drugs having less percentage of active constituents and are added to the genuine drug.

31. **Adulterants:** Adulterants are the substances purposefully added in original drug to increase profit in marketing and they look similar to original drug but do not contain any active chemical constituent.

32. **Barks:** Barks are the external tissues of stem.

33. **Fracture:** The transverse broken surface of the bark is known as fracture.

34. **Balsams (S. 00):** The oleoresins which contains benzoic acid or cinnamic acids are termed as balsams.

35. **Sialogogue:** The drugs which increases the secretion of saliva are called sialogogue, e.g. tobacco.

36. **Galactogogue:** The drug which increases the secretion of milk are called galactogogue, e.g. shatavari.

37. **Cholagogue:** The drug which increases secretion of bile, e.g. turmeric.

38. **Hydrogogue:** The drugs which promotes watery evacuation of the bowel are called as hydrogogue, e.g. jalap, calomel.

39. **Emmenagogue:** The substances which stimulates the menstrual flow are called as emmenagogue.

40. **Stomachics:** The substances which increases the secretion of gastric juice and the functional activity of stomach are called as stomachics, e.g. dill, fennel, coriander, gentian.

Q 1. How following scientists contributed in development of pharmacognosy?

1. Galen (S. 96, 98, 04, 05, 06, 07, 09; W. 98, 02)

- He was a Greek scientist.
- He found method of extraction.
- He developed "galenical pharmacy".
- Galenicals prepared are decoction, infusion.

2. Seydler (S. 97, 06, 09; W. 03, 06, 07, 08)

- He was a German scientist.
- He wrote the book "Pharmacognostica Gignostica".
- When he was a student, he published his thesis on "Sarspirella". The title of this thesis was "Analecta Pharmacognostica".
- He introduced the term "pharmacognosy" from two words:
  'Pharmakon' means a drug
  'Gnosis' means knowledge of.
- He explained the term as "knowledge of drugs".

3. Dioscoride (S. 05, 06, 08; W. 08)

- He was a Greek physician.
- He described several plants of medicinal importance.
- His book is "De Materia Medica".
- Materia medica is the text in which all natural products utilized by physicians were complied together to form materia medica giving their detailed information.

4. Hippocrates (S. 00, 06, 08, 09; W. 03, 06, 07)

- He was a Greek physician.
- He is known as "father of medicine".
- He has contributed to pharmacognosy by his study on "anatomy and physiology of human beings".

5. Aristotle (W. 03)

- He was a Greek philosopher.
- He explain his theory as a "Origin of Universe", the sun and earth.

- He studied the animal kingdom.
- He suggested the principle of classification of animals.

6. Sushruta (S. 09; W. 06)

- He was an Indian surgeon and physician.
- He knew about 1500 drugs.
- · He used to operate GIT.
- His collection is named as "Sushruta Samhita".

7. Charak (S. 96, 99, 04, 06, 07; W. 00, 01, 08)

- He was an Indian physician.
- He knew about 700 drugs.
- The drugs were obtained from plants and minerals.
- His collection is named as "Charak Samhita."

Scientists	Contribution
i. Galen	Extraction method
ii. Seydler	"Pharmacognostica Gignostica"
iii. Dioscoride	"De Materia Medica"
iv. Hippocrate	"Father of Medicine"
v. Aristotle	"Animal kingdom"/classification of animals.

Q 2. Give the scope of pharmacognosy. Explain history of pharmacognosy. (S. 96, 99, 00, 02; W. 96, 98, 99, 00, 01)

Scope of Pharmacognosy

- To provide knowledge of the natural plant and animal drugs.
- To provide knowledge of active constituents of drugs.
- To understand identification, extraction, purification, standardization and formulation of drugs.
- To find out adulteration in the drugs.
- Knowledge of pharmacognosy is useful in production of spices, cereals, paper, fabrics, paints, and also Bekari productions.

History of Pharmacognosy

- In Papyrus Ebers, an old documents, written in 1500 BC, Egyptions were aware of medicinal uses of several plants and animals and human anatomy also.
- The great Greek physician "Hippocrates" known as "father of medicine" studied the human anatomy and physiology.

- Aristotle philosopher is well known for his studies on "animal kingdom".
- Theophrastus is well known for study on "plant kingdom".
- Dioscoride, a Greek physician described several plants of medicinal importance in "De Materia Medica".
- Galen, a Greek scientist described the method of extraction of active constituent of crude drugs.
- Seydler, a German scientist, coined the term pharmacognosy in 1815 in his work entitled "Analecta Pharmacognostica".

Q 3. Write a note on "indigenous system of medicine" or "traditional Indian system of medicine" or "ancient system of medicine". (S. 98, 05, 07, 09; W. 96)

- Indian has rich heritage of large number of medicinal plants.
- These medicinal plants have been used for various medicinal purpose from many centuries.
- The different indigenous systems of medicines existing in India are:
  - i. Ayurveda
  - ii. Siddha
  - iii. Naturopathy
  - iv. Yoga
  - v. Unani.

i. Ayurveda (W. 07, 08)

Ayurveda is an oldest system of medicine prepared from two basic vedas, namely (i) Rigveda, (ii) Atharvaveda. The importance of this system is prevention of disease than treatment. Ayurveda includes diet specifications and importance of water purification. The dosage forms mentioned in Ayurveda are syrups, pills, powders. Pharmacopoeia of Ayurveda consists of more than 8000 species made up of natural drugs derived from minerals, herbals, animals and marine sources.

These are eight branches of Ayurveda:

- a. Kayachikitsa: Internal medicine.
- b. Tarkchikitsa: Psychological medicine.
- c. Kumar Bhritya: Paediatric medicines.
- d. Shalya Tantra: Surgery.
- e. Shalakya Tantra: Old age patients (geriatrics).
- f. Rasayana Tantra: ENT/Eye.

g. Agada Tantra: Toxicology (study of poisonous drugs).

h. Vajikaran Tantra: Aphrodiasics.

ii. Siddha/Siddhi (W. 06)

'Siddha' means achievements and practitioners of the method are known as 'siddhars'.

This method is originated in South India.

The material of siddha is mostly in Tamil language. "Siddhars" are saintly personalities who have studied medicine through a practice of Bhakti and Yoga. This system believes that all objects in universe are made up of five basic elements—earth, water, sky, fire and air. The identification of diseases is done through—pulse reading, colour of the body, study of voice, urine examination, status of digestive system and examination of tongue.

iii. Naturopathy (W. 00)

Naturopathy means use of components of nature in the treatment of diseases, i.e. naturopathy is based on laws of nature. Naturopathy gives importance to cleaning of physiological systems. It states that the disease can be completely treated by removing imbalance in internal and external atmosphere.

The diseases can be treated by using components of nature. Use of mud packs, baths and dietary controls are suggested in the naturopathy gives maximum importance to digestive system.

iv. Yoga (W. 00)

This system was practicised in routine in history of India.

- Yoga system gives importance to calmness to the brain and body.
- It gives physical and mental strength.
- One of the method of yoga is saving the physical energy.
- It focuses internal environment than external environment.
- This system gives importance to cardiovascular system and central nervous system. The main objectives of yoga are:
  a. Blood purification.
  b. Blood circulation.
  c. Tranquility.

v. Unani

This methodology is originated in India. This method suggest the use of plants and minerals mainly in natural forms.

Q 4. Differentiate between 'organised and unorganised drugs". (S. 97, 01, 05, 06, 07, 09; W. 98, 07, 08)

Organised drugs	Unorganised drugs
i. These are made up of cells.	i. These are made up of particles.
ii. They have definite size and shape.	ii. They do not have definite shape and size.
iii. Chemical constituents are present in the cells.	iii. Chemical constituents are present in the particles.
iv. Cellular arrangement is uniform in all the samples.	iv. Particle arrangement is changed from sample to sample.
v. Morphological study helps in identification of the drugs.	v. Morphological studies have less importance in identification of the drugs.
vi. Microscopical observations confirms the identification.	vi. Chemical tests confirms the identification.
vii. All the parts of the plants are organised.	vii. Plant exudates and plant extracts are unorganised in nature.
viii. The chemical constituents are formed during metabolism.	viii. The drugs are obtained by artificial process like injuries.
ix. The constituents are known as metabolic products.	ix. They are known as pathological products.
x. Example: Fennel, ginger	x. Example: Catechu, acacia

Q 5. What are pharmaceutical aids? Classify them with example. (S. 97, 98, 99, 02, 03, 06, 07, 08, 09; W. 98, 99, 01, 04, 06, 07)

Pharmaceutical Aids

The substances which are of little or no therapeutic value but essentially used in manufacture of or compounding of various pharmaceutical products are known as pharmaceutical aids.

Classification

a. *As per source*

• Plant source, e.g. acacia, fennel.
• Animal source, e.g. honey, beeswax.
• Mineral source, e.g. talc, kaolin.
• Synthetic source, e.g. glucose, fructose.

b. *As per application/use*

- Suspending agents, e.g. acacia, tragacanth.
- Emulsifying agents, e.g. acacia, beeswax.
- Thickening agents, e.g. starch, agar.
- Flavouring agents, e.g. coriander, cardamom.
- Sweetening agents, e.g. honey, glucose.
- Binding agents, e.g. starch, cellulose.
- Disintegrating agent, e.g. starch.
- Absorbent, e.g. kaolin.
- Diluent, e.g. lactose, glucose.
- Solvents, e.g. water, honey, arachis.
- Colouring agents, e.g. caramel, yellow oxide.

Q 6. Define technical products. Give examples.

Technical Products (W. 97)

The drugs which are used in the pharmaceutical industries are called as technical products.

i. Ginger is used in soft drinks and beverage.

ii. Caraway are used in bakeries.

iii. Catechu and Gambir are used in ink and dye industry and also in lather industries.

Technical Use (S. 96)

The use of drugs other than pharmaceutical use therapeutic use is called technical use.

CHAPTER 2

Classification of Crude Drugs

Q 1. What is the need/importance of classification of crude drugs?/Why the drugs are classified?/Give the object of classification of drugs. (S. 02)

Need of Classification

- It makes a simple study of drugs.
- Easy to study and remember properties of group of drugs.
- It saves the time.
- It is useful for effective use of knowledge.
- Huge number of drugs are in nature, it is very difficulty to study them separately.
- It gives correct and accurate information about the drug.
- To help in practical work.

Q 2. Enlist/name/state/give various methods/systems of classification of crude drugs. (S. 98, 99, 03; W. 96, 97, 98, 99, 01, 02)

- Alphabetical method.
- Taxonomical method.
- Morphological method/organoleptic method.
- Chemical method.
- Pharmacological method.
- Chemotaxonomical method.
- As per source.
- As per nature of drugs.

Q 3. Explain alphabetical method of classification of drugs. (S. 09)

Alphabetical Method

In this method, the drugs are mentioned alphabetically. This method is commonly used in preparing universal, official reference books.

Merits

- Useful method for books such as BP, BPC, USP, IP.
- Simple method.
- Location and tracing of drug is easy.
- Addition of drug is easy.
- No technical person is required for handling the system.

Demerits

- Original source is not clear by this classification.
- Scientific nature of drug cannot be identified by this method, whether the drug is organised or unorganised.

Q 4. Write in brief about toxonomical method of classification of drugs. (S. 09; W. 06)

Taxonomical Method

- This is a botanical type of classification.
- It is applicable to living organisms only (drugs obtained from plant, animals and microorganisms).
- Taxonomy helps in systematic classification of living organisms.
- In this method various steps are taken for proper classification.
- Each step indicates certain characters:
    i. Kingdom
    ii. Subkingdom
    iii. Phylum
    iv. Subphylum
    v. Class
    vi. Subclass
    vii. Division
    viii. Order
    ix. Family
    x. Genus
    xi. Species

Merits

- It helps in determining scientific name of living organism.
- It explains some characters of plants.

Demerits/Limitations

- Nonliving drugs cannot be classified.

- If characters of two families are very close then classification become difficult.
- Technical person is required for classification of drugs.

Q 5. Describe the chemotaxonomical method of classification of crude drugs.

- It is the latest method which brings together advantages of chemical method and taxonomical method.
- This method gives details of taxonomy (family) and active chemical constituent of the drug.
- For example:
  i. Ginger can be explained as:
  Biological source: Ginger is obtained from rhizomes of zingiber officinale.
  Family: Zingiberaceae.
  Chemical constituents: It contains not less than 2% of volatile oil.
  ii. Nux vomica
  Biological source: It is obtained from dried, seeds of Strychnos nux vomica.
  Family: Ligniaceae.
  Chemical constituents: It contains not less than 1.2% of strychnine.

Merits
- It gives information of family and chemical constituents.
- It is scientific method.
- It also gives information about 1% of chemical constituent presence in the drug.

Demerits
Skilled and qualified person is required for classification of drugs.

Q 6. Discuss chemical method of classification of crude drugs. (S. 96, 05, 06, 09; W. 98)

Chemical Method of Classification
- In this method the drugs are classified according to the nature of active chemical constituent present in the drug.
- Active chemical constituents are mainly responsible for physiological or pharmacological actions.
- The method of classification is as follows:
  i. Carbohydrates, e.g. starch, honey.

ii. Proteins, e.g. gelatin, wool.
iii. Lipids, e.g. arachis oil, beeswax
iv. Vitamins, e.g. cod liver oil, shark liver oil.
v. Enzymes, e.g. yeast, papaine.
vi. Tannins, e.g. catechu.
vii. Resins, e.g. asafoetida, myrrh.
viii. Alkaloids, e.g. cinchona, ipecac.
ix. Glycosides, e.g. digitalis, aloe.
x. Volatile oils, e.g. fennel, coriander.
xi. Gums, e.g. acacia.
xii. Mucilages, e.g. agar, tragacanth.

Merits

- Chemical constituents are known.
- Medicinal uses are known.
- It explains physical and chemical properties of active constituent.
- It helps in extraction process during selection of menstruum.
- It gives information about pharmacological action of drug.
- Helpful for identification of mainly unorganised drugs.
- It helps in proper storage of drugs.

Demerits

- If drug contains two or more constituents, then it is difficult to classify.
- Drugs of different origin may grouped under similar chemical title.
- The technical person having the knowledge of chemical constituents is necessary.
- Variations in the % of chemical constituents may confuse during classification.
- Adulterated drugs may misguide during classification.

Q 7. Explain pharmacological method of classification of crude drugs. Give its merits and demerits. (S. 06, 07, 09; W. 04, 07, 08)

Pharmacological Method of Classification

- In this method drugs are classified as per pharmacological action or physiological action of active constituent.
- It should be noted that some drugs may produce more than one pharmacological effects and then classification become more complex.

- In this method the drugs are classified as per actions and uses:
  i. Carminative, e.g. coriander, clove.
  ii. Purgatives, e.g. senna, castor oil.
  iii. Cardiotonics, e.g. digitalis, squill.
  iv. CNS stimulants, nux vomica.
  v. Diuretics, e.g. gokharu, purarnava.
  vi. Oxytocics, e.g. ergot.
  vii. Antimalarials, cinchona.
  viii. Anticancer, e.g. vinca.
  ix. Antirheumatics, e.g. guggul, colchicum.
  x. Bitters, e.g. Cinchona, Gention.
  xi. Antidysenteric, e.g. ipecacuhna.

Merits/Advantages

- Nature of physiological action can be understood.
- Nature of pharmacological action can be understood.
- Gives exact idea about the storage and uses of drug.
- Medicinal uses are understood.
- The drugs whose chemical constituents are not known can be classified.

Demerits/Limitations

- Difficult to classify the drug showing many pharmacological actions.
- Does not give idea about chemistry of chemical constituent.
- No idea about mechanism of action of drug.
- Does not give idea about doses of drugs.
- In classification adverse (–ve) effects are not mentioned.
- Do not give idea about morphology of a drug.
- Knowledge of pharmacology is required for classification of drugs.
- Contraindications of drugs are not mentioned thus may produce dangerous effects.

Q 8. Describe morphological/organoleptic method of classification of crude drugs. (S. 99, 04, 08; W. 99, 00, 06)

Morphological/Organoleptic Classification

In this method the drugs are classified according to the parts of plant (drug) like leaves, fruits, flowers, woods, barks, extracts, gums, etc.

Parts of Plants

- *Barks*: Arjuna, cinchona.
- *Flowers*: Clove, saffron.
- *Leaves*: Senna, digitalis.
- *Fruits*: Fennel, coriander.
- *Seeds*: Nux vomica, linseed.
- *Rhizome*: Ginger.
- *Stems*: Vasaka.
- *Flowering tops*: Tulsi.
- *Bulbs*: Garlic.
- *Tubers*: Aconite.

Merits

- It gives an idea about the morphological characters of drugs.
- It is a convenient method for students for practical purposes.
- Addition of drugs in system is easy.
- Location and tracing of drug is easy.
- Adulterant can be identified easily.
- Method is helpful in deciding purity of drug.
- It gives idea about chemical constituents/composition of drug, e.g. leaves, rhizomes, tubers contains starch.

Disadvantages/Demerits

- Does not give an idea about biological sources and uses of drugs.
- The drugs which do not have exact morphological form cannot be classified by this method.
- When different parts of plant contain different chemical constituents, it is difficult to classify them.
- The method is applicable to entire crude drug only.
- The quantity of drug required for classification is more.

CHAPTER 3

Systematic Study of Drugs
(Scheme of Pharmacognostic Studies)

Q 1. Explain the terms in short.

1. Title/Official Title (Official Source) (S. 96; W. 00)

- Title is the official name of the drug.
- It is the name of drug mentioned in official books like IP, BP, NF, etc.
- The title is in English or Latin.
- The title is always written in capital letters.
- In various pharmacopoeia different titles of the same drugs may be suggested.
- Examples: Ginger, Catechu, Fennel.

2. Synonyme (W. 03)

- Synonymes are the alternative names of the drug.
- Synonymes are in regional languages.
- They are used in specific geographical areas.
- Pharmacopoeia of India recognises synonymes in English and Hindi languages.
- Synonyme helps in collecting information available in various regions.
- Examples: Ginger.
  Synonyms: Adrak (Hindi)
  　　　　　 Ale (Marathi).

3. Geographical Source

- It informs the geographical places where the plants or animals occurs naturally and where the drug is obtained commercially.

- It helps in knowing atmospheric conditions required for the plants and animals.

4. Biological Source (Biological Origin) (S. 96)

- The drug can be obtained from plant source or animal source which is named as biological source. It may be of two types:
  - i. *Botanical source*: It means drug is obtained from plant, e.g. arjuna consist of dried stem bark of the plant known as "Terminalia arjuna".
  - ii. *Animal source*: It means drug is obtained from animals, e.g. shark liver oil is obtained from shark fish.
- Importance of biological source: It gives information about:
  - i. Source—plant/animal.
  - ii. Parts of plant/animal.
  - iii. Maturity state of parts of plants.
  - iv. Scientific name of plant/animal.
  - v. Method of collection of drug.
  - vi. Family and scientific name of the drug.
  - vii. Pharmacopoeial standards.

5. Collection

- It gives information about process of collection of parts of plant and prevention of damage to the plant during collection.
- The collection gives knowledge of their chemical constituents responsible for therapeutic action.
- Collection is considered for its purity of drugs.
- Generally the plants are collected when they are rich in their chemical constituents.
- The drugs containing thermolabile substances and volatile oils are collected at low temperature.
- Thus, choice of collection depends upon the chemical constituents of the plants.

6. Cultivation

- It explains agricultural aspects.
- It explains scientific process of cultivation of plants.
- Cultivation means a systematic reproduction of plant.
- It informs about:
  - i. Method of reproduction of plant.

ii. Required rainfall and water supply.

iii. Nature of soil to be used.

iv. Fertilizers required.

v. Plant protection involves used of insecticides.

vi. Mechanical methods, e.g. cutting, scraping, burning, etc.

• Cultivation helps in complete growth of plant and it maximizes active chemical constituent of the drug.

7. Preparation of Drugs for Market

It includes various steps like removal of unwanted parts of plants, drying, packing and transportation.

8. Morphology/Morphological Characters (Organoleptic Characters)

• It is also known as macroscopy.

• Morphology means the study of external characters or parts of the plants.

• The external characters or sensory characters of the plant are known as morphological characters or organoleptic characters.

• Observations like appearance, surface, size, shape, colour odour, taste are taken with sensory organs hence are also known as organoleptic characters.

9. Microscopy/Microscopical Characters (Histological Characters) (W. 00)

• Microscopy involves the study of microscopical features such as TS, LS and observed under microscope.

• The characters which are observed under microscope are called microscopic characters/histological characters.

• The specific microscopic characters such as stomata, trichomes, starch grains helps in evaluation of drugs.

10. Chemical Constituent/Active Constituent/Active Principle (S. 96)

It means main constituent of the drug which produce a therapeutic action.

• A drug may contain many chemical constituents.

• Some of the chemical constituents are capable of producing physiological and pharmacological actions on human body and other animals. Some drugs contains several constituents which are inert.

- The unorganised drugs are identified and confirmed by chemical constituents.
- *Example*: Cinnamon

  Chemical constituents
    i. Volatile oils
    ii. Tannins
    iii. Mucilages
       - Volatile oil is the main chemical constituents.
       - The mucilage and tannins are inactive constituents.

11. Substitute/Substituent

- Substituents are the alternative varieties of the drugs having less percentage of active constituents and are added to genuine drug.
- Substitutes are the unwanted parts of the plant present in original drug like leaf or roots of the same plants and sometimes other variety of drugs are mixed in the original drug.
- *Examples*:
    i. *Senna*: Substitutes—dog senna, Japanese senna.
    ii. *Digitalis leaf*: Substitutes—other parts of digitalis plant looking similar to that of digitalis leaf or digitalis lanata variety.

12. Adulterants

Adulterants are the substances purposefully added in original drug to increase profit in marketing and they look similar to original drug but does not contain any active constituent.

- The process of worthless admixtures in the genuine is known as adulteration.
- Adulterated mixture may prove dangerous to the patients.
- Adulteration is profit oriented process.
- Powders and oil can be easily adulterated.
- Adulterants are sometimes similar to genuine drug in respect of morphological characters such as size, shape, small, etc. but do not have any chemical constituents.
- *Example*
    i. The seeds of strychonus nux vomica are adulterated with that of "strychonus blanda" which do not contains strychnine.
    ii. Ginger is adulterated with exhausted ginger.

13. Uses

Uses of drugs means the actual physiological and pharmacological effects produced by drug on human body and other animals.

- *Therapeutic uses/pharmacological uses*: It means use of drugs in the treatment of diseases or disorders.
- *Pharmaceutical uses*: When a drug is used for other purposes that its medicinal use, they are commonly known as pharmaceutical uses (technical uses), e.g. fennel, ginger as flavouring agents and turmeric as colouring agents.

CHAPTER 4

Collection and Preparation of Crude Drugs for Market

Q 1. Explain the term "collection" in the preparation of crude drugs for market?

Collection of Crude Drugs

- Collection gives information about the process of collection of parts of plant and prevention of damage to the plant during collection.
- The collection gives knowledge of their chemical constituents responsible for therapeutic actions.
- Collection is considered for its purity.
- Choice of collection of drugs depends upon type of chemical constituents of plant.
- Generally the plants are collected when they are rich in their chemical constituents.
- The drugs containing thermolabile substances and volatile oils are collected at low temperature.
- The collection of drug may involve the maximum concentration of active constituent.
- Collection should be done in a proper environmental conditions.

Examples

- The drugs which constitute the leaf and flowering tops of the plants are collected just before they reach their flowering stage, e.g. senna, digitalis, belladona.
- The barks are generally collected in spring environment, i.e. in the early summer.
- The fruits are collected depending upon the parts of fruit which are pharmaceutically important.

- Rhizomes are collected after full vegetative growth of the plant.
- The unorganised drugs such as gums, resins are collected as soon as they ooze out of the plant.

Q 2. Explain "garbling/dressing" in preparation of crude drugs for market.

Garbling/Dressing

"Garbling is the process in which there is a removal of soil, dirt and foreign organic parts of the same plant or nonconstituting drug."
- Garbling is the next step in the preparation of crude drug for market after drying.
- If such foreign material is permitted in the crude drugs, the quality of drug will be reduced. Hence, the percentage of foreign material should be such that it should passes the pharmacopoeial limits.

Examples

- Drugs constituting rhizomes are separated carefully from roots or rootlets and also from stem bases.
- The pieces of iron must be removed with magnet in cases of castor seeds before crushing and by shifting.
- The pieces of bark should be removed by peeling in processing of gum acacia.
- The excessive stems in case of lobelia and stramonium are needed to be removed.

Importance of Garbling

- It improves quality of drug.
- It improves purity of drug.
- It gives shining appearance to the drug.
- It increases stability of drug.
- Garbling increases market value of the product.

Q 3. Explain "drying" in preparation of crude drugs for market. (S. 96, 07)

Drying

Drying means complete removal of water from the drugs.
- Before marketing a crude drug, it is necessary to dry the drug to get a good pharmaceutical appearance to the drugs.
- Drying should be done without loss of chemical constituents.

- Drying consists of removal of sufficient moisture content of crude drug. So as to improve its quality and to prevent growth of microorganisms.
- Drying also inhibits partially the enzyme reactions.
- The slicing, cutting into small pieces is done to increase the rate of drying.

Types of drying

- Natural drying.
- Artificial drying:
  - i. Tray dryers
  - ii. Vacuum dryers
  - iii. Spray dryers.

1. *Natural Drying/Sun Drying*

- It may be either direct sundrying or drying in the shade.
- If the natural colour of drug and the volatile principles of the drugs are to be retained, then drying in shade is preferred.
- If the contents of the drugs are quite stable to temperature and sunlight, then the drugs can be dried directly in sunlight.

2. *Artificial Drying*

It is done by using following devices.

  - i. *Tray dryers* (*an oven*): The drugs which do not contain volatile oils and are quite stable to heat are dried in tray dryers.
  - ii. *Vacuum dryers*: The drugs which are sensitive to higher temperatures, are dried by this process, e.g. tannic acid, digitalis leaves.
  - iii. *Spray drying*: Some drugs which are highly sensitive to atmospheric conditions and also to temperature of vacuum drying are dried by spray drying method, e.g. papaya latex, pectin, tannins are dried by spray drying.

Q 4. Explain "harvesting" in the preparation of crude drugs for market.

- Harvesting is an important operation in the cultivation technology.
- Harvesting can be done correctly by skilled workers.
- It is a hard job and may not be economical.
- In some cases, the harvesting may be done by mechanical devices.

- The underground drugs like roots, rhizomes, tubers, etc. are harvested by mechanical devices such as diggers or the lifters.
- The tubers and roots are thoroughly washed in water to remove earthy matter.
- Many times flowers, seeds and small fruits are harvested by a special device known as a seed strippers.
- The technique of beating the plant with bamboos is used in case of cloves.
- The cochineal insects are collected from branches of cactus by brushing.
- Fennel, coriander and caraway plants are uprooted and dried. After drying either they are thrashed or beaten and the fruits are separated by winnowing.

Q 5. Explain "packing" in the preparation of crude drugs for market.

- "Packing" is a technique in which drug is packed in a container which protects the drug from contamination.
- The climatic conditions during transportation and storage should be considered while packing the drugs.
- Packing improves quality and stability of the drugs.

Examples

- Colophony and balsam of tolu are packed in kerosene tin.
- Asafoetida is stored in well closed containers to prevent loss of volatile oils.
- Cod liver oil is very sensitive to sunlight hence it should be stored in light resistant containers.
- The drugs which are very sensitive to moisture and are costly, should be packed very carefully in airtight containers, e.g. digitalis, ergot.
- The drugs like roots, seeds and others which do not need special attention are packed in gunny bags. While in some cases bags are coated with polythene internally.
- Packing also protects the drug from damage during transportation.

Q 6. Give the method of cultivation and collection of "senna" leaf. (S. 00, 01, 02; W. 98, 06)

Cultivation

- The senna plants are cultivated by sowing the seeds.

- The seeds are mixed with sand before cultivation.
- The sowing of seed can be carried out in the month of March, April or November, December.

Requirements

- Soil should have water nonretaining property and should be red and black colour.
- The rainfall should be heavy about 1500 to 3000 mm/year.
- Temperature should be warm about 25°C average temperature.

Process

- The seeds are sown in nursery beds.
- They germinate within 3 weeks.
- After germination within 15 days, the young plants are transferred into farms.

Collection

- The plants are allowed to grow for 3–5 months.
- The flowering tops are cut off periodically to ensure maximum branching.
- When the leaflets have measurable thickness in the month of September or February the leaves are manually collected.

Other Processes

- The leaflets are subjected to harvesting.
- In the process, large pieces of stems, flowers, seeds are rejected.
- The leaflets are spread on floor and dried in shelves.
- A care is taken that overlapping of leaflets is avoided during drying.
- The leaflets loose about 50–60% of their weights.
- Yellowish green coloured leaves are selected.
- They are packed in gunny bags under pressure and marketed.

Q 7. What are the methods of cultivation and collection of digitalis leaves? (S. 96, 97, 99, 03, 07, 08; W. 05, 08)

Digitalis Leaves

Cultivation

It needs sandy, light soil, rich in calcium and traces of magnesium. Rain fall about 1500 mm/year. Average temperature of 15°C.

Process

- Soil is sterilized by steam before sowing the seeds.
- Seeds are mixed with fine sand and sown in nursery beds in the month of March or April.
- Two to three weeks are required for germination.
- The young plants are transplanted in the month of September to November.
- The area under cultivation is kept free from weeds.

Collection

- In the first year, the plants bears rosette leaves and in the second year sessile leaves.
- The plant flowers in the month of April and is followed by fruiting.
- Before that the leaves are manually collected in afternoon hours.
- If the plants are to be allowed to grow, the flowering tops are removed.

Other processes

- The digitalis leaves are immediately taken to drying centre.
- Leaves are spread on the trays with fine wire netting bottom.
- They are dried in vaccum dryers.
- The temperature of drying is maintained below 60°C and continued till leaves contains moisture less than 5%.
- The leaves are packed in airtight containers along with suitable dehydrating agent.

Q 8. What are the methods of cultivation and collection of opium? (W. 02, 04)

Opium

Cultivation

- Cultivation of opium is controlled and monitored by government of India.

Requirements

- Soil water nonretaining grey or whitish coloured.
- Temperature: Average temperature is 35°C.
- Rainfall: About 100 mm/year.

Process of Cultivation

- Cultivation is carried out by sowing the seeds.
- The seeds are mixed with sand and scattered on the land.
- Distance between two plant to be maintained is about 25 cm.
- The seeds are germinated within two weeks.

Collection

- In the month of February or March in the afternoon or evening hours the vertical incisions are taken.
- The incisions are taken from top to bottom of the fruit.
- Three to four incisions are taken at a time.
- Whitish latex comes out of fruits in early morning.
- Using a blade, latex is collected.
- Latex is dried and packed as per the norms stated by government of India.
- For transportation and marketing along with possession of the drug, appropriate licences are required.

Q 9. Give the method of cultivation and collection of Rauwolfia. (W. 00, 01, 07)

Rauwolfia

Cultivation

- The plants grows in wide ranges of atmospheric conditions.
- Soil should be rich in clay and water nonretaining.
- The pH of soil should be 4.
- Temperature of about 10 to 38°C.
- Rainfall: 250 to 500 mm.

Process of cultivation

- Plants are propogated using sexual method as well as vegetative method.
- The seeds are sown after selecting healthy seeds into nursery beds.
- Sowing is carried out in the month of May and June.
- The young plants are transferred into the forms in August or September.
- Distance between two plants should be about 30 cm.
- In vegetative method root cuttings are used.

- The plants are provided with chemical fertilizers like urea and ammonium sulphate.

Collection

- When the plants are about 3 to 4 years old, they are uprooted.
- The stem bases are separated.
- The roots are washed and dried in air.
- Then they are packed and marketed.

Q 10. What are the methods of cultivation and collection of ergot? (S. 09)

Ergot

Cultivation

- Ergot is a fungus.
- Some part of the life cycle of the fungus is completed in soil of air and another part is of life cycle is completed on rye plant.
- The fungus growth can be developed artificially.
- Ascospores are developed in a nutrient medium.
- The colonies are collected and diluted with H_2O.
- The solution is spread over rye plant.
- The sclerotia produced, fall on the grounds and they are collected.

Collection

- The collection is either manual process or mechanical process.
- They are placed in 30% solution of NaCl.
- The matured and well developed sclerotia float on the surface.
- After collection sclerotia are dried thoroughly and stored in dark coloured containers along with suitable dehydrating agent and marketed.

CHAPTER 5

Chemical Nature of Natural Drugs
(Alkaloids, Glycosides, Tannins, Resins, Vitamins, etc.)

Q 1. Define alkaloids. Classify alkaloids giving suitable examples. (S. 00, 01, 02, 04, 09; W. 98, 05)

Alkaloids

The alkaloids are basic nitrogenous organic products of plant origin, having marked physiological actions when administered internally.

Classification of Alkaloids

Alkaloids are divided into two main classes:

a. *Nonheterocyclic alkaloids*: Ephedrine (ephedra), colchicine (colchicum).

b. *Heterocyclic alkaloids*:

Types of alkaloids	Examples	Source
1. Tropane	Atropine	Datura
2. Quinoline	Quinine	Cinchona
3. Indole	Strychnine	Nux-vomica
4. Isoquinoline	Papaverine	Opium
5. Phenanthrene	Morphine	Opium
6. Purine	Caffeine	Tea
7. Pyrrole and pyrolidine	Nicotine	Tobacco
8. Pyridine and piperidine	Lobeline	Lobela
9. Imidazole	Pilocarpine	Pilocarpus
10. Terpenoid	Aconitine	Aconite

Q 2. Give the properties and role of alkaloids in plants. (S. 08; W. 96)

Properties of Alkaloids

• Alkaloids are colourless, solid and crystalline.

- Alkaloids are insoluble in water but soluble in organic solvents.
- Alkaloids in the salt form are water soluble and insoluble in organic solvents.
- Alkaloids are optically active being usually levorotatory.
- Alkaloids are highly potent medicaments and posses curative properties.
- Alkaloids are biosynthesized due to participation of several amino acids and enzymatic systems.

Role of Alkaloids in Plants (W. 08)

- Alkaloids are nitrogenous organic compounds.
- Alkaloids are basic in nature and so they can react with acid molecules easily.
- Alkaloids are metabolic products and so they are produced, stored and utilized whenever necessary.
- The plants considers alkaloid molecules as source of nitrogen atom. They are utilized in protein synthesis and synthesis hormones.
- The alkaloids are generally associated with acids and so they can act as carriers of acid molecules.
- The alkaloids helps in maintenance of regular physiological activities like growth and reproduction.
- The alkaloids are protective agents.
- The alkaloids are detoxicating agents.
- If total amount of alkaloids present in the plant is removed, the plant is not affected at all.
- Amount of alkaloids change from time to time in a day and from season to season in an year.

Q 3. Explain various chemical tests for alkaloids. (S. 98, 99, 00, 01, 02, 03, 04, 06, 07; W. 96, 98, 01, 07)

Chemical Tests for Alkaloids

Precipitation Tests

- *Mayer's test*: Alkaloids gives cream or pale yellow precipitate with Mayer's reagent (potassium mercuric iodide solution).
- *Dragendorff's test*: Alkaloids gives brown or reddish brown coloured precipitate with Dragendorff's reagent (potassium bismuth iodide solution).
- *Wagner's test*: Alkaloids gives brown or reddish brown coloured precipitate with Wagner's reagent (iodine and potassium iodide solution).

- *Hager's test*: Alkaloids with Hager's reagent gives yellow precipitate (saturated solution of picric acid).

Q 4. Give the general methods of extraction of alkaloids. (S. 02, 09; W. 98, 04)

Extraction Method of Alkaloids

The objective of extraction process is to separate alkaloid molecules from all other molecules.

Laboratory Method of Extraction of Alkaloids

- The drug sample is powdered.
- The sample is treated with strong base (NaOH).
- The added base reacts with acid molecules present along with alkaloids.
- The products formed are neutralized products, i.e. salt and water.
- The salts formed are soluble in water, so the mixture is washed with H_2O. It forms aqueous phase. The alkaloid molecules get isolated from aqueous phase.
- A small quantity of any suitable organic solvents are added 4 to 5 times. The organic solvents dissolves the alkaloid, molecules in it.
- Now in the mixture there are two phases—aqueous phase and organic phase. These two phases can be separated using suitable apparatus like separating funnel.
- The organic phase is collected in evaporating dish.
- After heating the organic solvent get evaporated and residue of alkaloid is obtained.

Nowadays extraction can be done by using chromatography technique.

Q 5. Give the therapeutic effects/uses/applications of alkaloids. (W. 99)

Alkaloids are highly potent medicaments and posses curative properties.

- It have narcotic action, e.g. morphine.
- It have tranquillizer action, e.g. reserpine.
- It is a nerve stimulant, e.g. strychnine.
- It is a local anaesthetic, e.g. cinchocaine, cocaine.
- It is an antispasmodic, e.g. atropine.
- It is a CNS stimulant, e.g. caffeine.
- It is a antimalaria, e.g. quinine.

Q 6. What are glycosides? How are they classified? (S. 00, 01, 05, 09; W. 99, 08)

Glycosides

Glycosides are organic compounds which on hydrolysis give one or more molecules of sugar of one nonsugar molecule. Sugar molecule is called glycon and nonsugar molecule is called aglycone or genin.

$$\text{Glycoside} \xrightarrow{\text{Hydrolysis}} \underset{\text{(Glycon)}}{\text{Sugar}} + \underset{\text{(Aglycone)}}{\text{Nonsugar}}$$

Classification of Glycosides

a. Depending upon Glycone Present

Glucose $\longrightarrow$ Glucoside

Fructose $\longrightarrow$ Fructoside

Rhamnose $\longrightarrow$ Rhamnoside

b. As per Linkage

- C-glycosides: Carbon linkage, e.g. sennosides in senna.
- O-glycosides: Flavone glycosides, e.g. amygdalin in bitter almond.
- N-glycosides, e.g. sinigrin in black mustard.
- S-glycosides, e.g. prunassin in wild cherry bark.

c. As per Chemical Nature of Aglycone

- Cyanogenetic glycosides: On hydrolysis gives one of molecule of H, C, N, e.g. Prunassin in wild cherry.
- Saponin glycosides: Forms soap solution in water, e.g. glycerrhizine in glycerrhiza.
- Cardiac glycosides: Digitoxigenin.
- Thiocyanate glycosides, e.g. sinigrin.
- Phenolic glycosides, e.g. salicin, rhein.
- Steroidal glycosides, e.g. digitalis glycosides.

d. As per Pharmacological Method

- Cardiotonics, e.g. digitalis.
- Laxative, e.g. senna.
- Bitter tonics, e.g. picrorrhiza.
- Expectorants, e.g. glycerrhiza.

Q 7. Define and classify volatile oils giving suitable examples. Give the properties and uses of volatile oils. (S. 98, 99, 05, 08; W. 06, 07)

Volatile oils are odours volatile principles of plant and animal sources which are easily evaporable.

Classification of Volatile Oils

- Alcohol containing volatile oils, e.g. pepermint, cardamom.
- Aldehyde containing volatile oils, e.g. cinnamon, lemon, orange.
- Hydrocarbon containing volatile oils, e.g. turpentine.
- Ketone containing volatile oils, e.g. caraway.
- Oxide containing volatile oils, e.g. eucalyptus.
- Phenolic-ester containing volatile oils, e.g. fennel, Nutmeg.
- Phenol containing volatile oils, e.g. clove.

General Properties of Volatile Oils

- They have characteristic odour.
- They have high retractive index.
- Most of volatile oils are optically active.
- They are either colourless rarely coloured.
- They have aromatic taste.
- They are insoluble in water and soluble in ether, alcohol, etc.
- They have good essence. The oils are called essence oils.

Uses of Volatile Oils

- As flavouring agents and perfumes.
- As carminatives.
- As stomachic.
- Externally, counter irritant.
- As a spices.
- As a local anaesthetics.

Q 8. Differentiate between fixed oils and volatile oils. (S. 96, 04, 08; W. 02)

Difference

Fixed oils	Volatile oils
i. These are thick, viscous, coloured liquid with characteristic odour.	i. These are thin with charac teristic od

Contd.

Fixed oils	Volatile oils
ii. They are nonvolatile and cannot be distilled.	ii. They are volatile and can be distilled.
iii. They can be saponified.	iii. They cannot be saponified.
iv. Becomes rancid.	iv. Does not becomes rancid.
v. Gives permanent stain.	v. Does not give permanent stain.
vi. They are edible.	vi. Generally, they are not edible.
vii. Does not evaporate.	vii. When exposed, it evaporates.
viii. They are the compounds related to fatty acids.	viii. They are compounds of alcohol.
ix. Examples: Castor oil, arachis oil.	ix. Examples: Clove oil, eucalyptus oil.

Q 9. Definte tannins. Classify tannins giving suitable examples. (S. 97, 00, 05, 07; W. 98)

Tannins are the derivatives of polyhydroxy benzoic acid and are capable of precipitating proteins.

Classification of Tannins

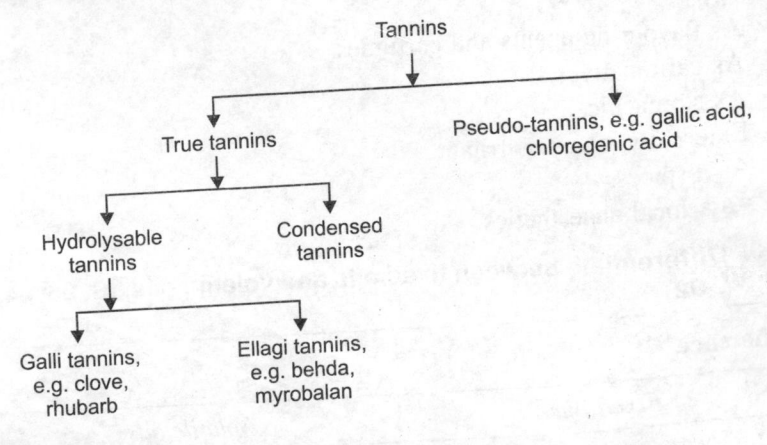

I. True Tannins

...us compounds soluble in water having high

i. *Hydrolysable Tannins*

These types of tannins can be hydrolysed with the help of mineral acids (HCl, HNO_3, H_2SO_4) hence called hydrolysable tannins. They are of two types:

a. *Galli tannins*: The hydrolysis product is gallic acid, e.g. clove, rhubarb.

b. *Ellagi tannins*: The hydrolysis product is ellagic acid, e.g. behda, myrobalan.

ii. *Condensed Tannins*

They cannot be hydrolysed. If they are subjected for hydrolysis, the molecules break downs and the decomposition product "phlobaphene" is obtained and so they are known as phlobatannins.

Phlobaphene is insoluble in water and red in colour, e.g. catechu.

II. Pseudo-tannins

These are tannin like substances having low molecular weights, e.g. gallic acid, chlorgenic acid.

Q 10. Give the properties, uses and chemical tests for tannins. (S. 96, 97; W. 01)

Properties of Tannins

- Tannins are soluble in water, dilute alkalies, alcohol, glycerine.
- Tannins are insoluble in other organic solvents.
- Tannins have a bitter and astringent in taste.
- Tannins combines with skin proteins and precipitates them.
- On hydrolysis by enzymes, tannins decompose mainly into glucose and gallic acid.

Uses of Tannins (S. 09)

- As astringents.
- Causes contraction of smooth muscles.
- Used in leather industry, inks and dyes.
- Used in food processing, food ripening and in manufacturing of tea, cocoa.
- In treatment of mouth and throat infections.

General Chemical Tests for Tannins (S. 07; W. 04)

1. *Gold beater skin test*: A piece of gold beaters skin (membrane of intestine of ox) + 2% dilute HCl, wash with distilled water. Add

tannin solution. Allow it to react for 5 minutes Add 1% ferrous sulphate solution.
- *Observation*: Brown to black colour shows positive test for tannins.

2. *Phenazone test*: 5 ml of aqueous drug extract + 0.9 gm sodium acid phosphate ($NaHPO_4$), warm, cool, filter to get filtrate.
Add 2% phenazone solution $\rightarrow$ coloured precipitate is observed.

3. *Catechin test*: Take drug extract of tannin solution and boil a dip match stick in it. Dry in air. Add a drop of concentration of HCl $\rightarrow$ purple or violet coloured is observed (condensed tannins).

4. Tannins with aqueous $FeCl_3$ solution gives blue, black or green colour.

5. Tannins, when treated with 1% gelatin soluiton and 10% NaCl solution, a precipitate is observed.

Q 11. What are resins? Classify resins with suitable examples, mention the properties of resins? (S. 96, 00, 05, 06; W. 01, 02, 04, 07)

Resins

Resins are amorphous, translucent solids or semisolids or liquid substances usually obtained as an exudate from plants.

Resins are either metabolic or pathological products.

Classification of Resins

Depending upon the functional group present, resins are classified as:
- Acid resins, e.g. colophony, myrrh.
- Ester resins, e.g. benzoin, storax.
- Resin alcohols, e.g. balsam of Peru.
- Mixed resins (resin Combinations):
    i. Gum-resins, e.g. Canada balsam.
    ii. Oleo-resins e.g. capsicum (combination of volatile oil and resin).
    iii. Oleo-gum-resin, e.g. asafoetida, guggul.
    iv. Glycoresins: Combination of sugar and resin.
    v. Balsams: They are the derivatives of acids like benzoic acid and cinnamic acid, e.g. balsam of peru, balsam of Tolu.

General Properties of Resins
- Amorphous in nature.
- Insoluble in water.

- They are end products of metabolism.
- On heating they soften and finally melt.
- Dissolve in alcohol, chloroform and ether.
- Burn with characteristic smoky flame.

Q 12. Differentiate between 'resin' and 'oleogum resins'.

Resins	Oleogum Resins
i. These are amorphous products of complex chemical nature	i. These are basically resins
ii. Chemically they are mixtures of resin acids, resin alcohols	ii. Chemically they consist of volatile oil, gum and resins
iii. Example: Storax	iii. Example: Asafoetida myrrh

Q 13. Define and classify carbohydrates giving suitable examples.

Carbohydrates

Carbohydrates are polyhydroxy aldehydes or polyhydroxy ketones or compounds which on hydrolysis gives either of above.

Classification

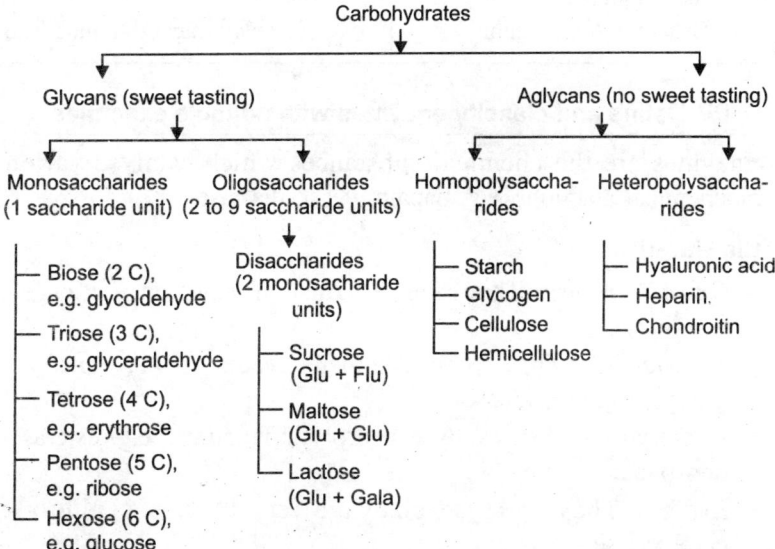

Q 14. Write a note on 'gums' and 'mucilages'.

Gums

Gums are pathological products formed after any injury to the plant.

- The plants containing schizogenous ducts or glands can form the gums.
- These ducts or glands forms and eliminates sticky, semiliquids.
- These substances prevent entry of microbes through injured area.
- The process of formation and deposition of gum is known as "gummosis" and the products as gums.
- Examples: Acacia gum, guar gum.

Mucilages

Mucilages are physiological products and can be obtained along with gums or any other constituents, e.g. tragacanth mucilage.

Gums	Mucilages
i. Gums are translucent and amorphous substances	i. Mucilages are plant products
ii. These are plant exudates	ii. These are present in the cell.
iii. These are pathological products	iii. These are normal products
iv. No red colour with ruthenium red	iv. Red colour with ruthenium red
v. Example: Acacia gum	v. Example: Tragacanth mucilage

Q 15. Define and classify enzymes with suitable examples.

Enzymes are the chemical substances which catalyse various biochemical reactions, e.g. papain, yeast, diastase.

Classification

- *Oxido-reductases*: They catalyze oxidation-reduction reaction, e.g. tyrosinase.
- *Transferases*: They catalyse transfer reactions, i.e. transfer of groups, e.g. hexokinase.
- *Hydrolyases*: They catalyse hydrolytic reactions, e.g. esterases, phosphatase.
- *Lyases:* They catalyse cleavage reactions, e.g. aldolase, carboxylase.

- *Isomerases*: They catalyse isomerization reactions, e.g. epimerase.
- *Ligases*: These enzymes catalyse the formation of bond, e.g. DNA ligase.

Q 16. Define and classify vitamins giving suitable examples.

Vitamins

Vitamins are the organic compounds which are found in natural food stuffs and essential for normal growth and metabolic functions of the body.

Classification

- *Fat soluble vitamins*: Vitamins A, D, E, and K.
- *Water soluble vitamins*:
  - i. Vitamin C (ascrobic acid)
  - ii. Vitamin B complex group:
    - – Thiamine (B_1)
    - – Riboflavin (B_2)
    - – Niacin (B_3)
    - – Pyridoxin (B_6)
    - – Pantothenic acid
    - – Biotin
    - – Folic acid
    - – Lipolic acid (PABA)
    - – Cyanocobalamin (vitamin B_{12}).

Q 17. Write a note on perfumes and flavouring agents. (W. 03)

Perfumes and Flavouring Agents

Perfumes (Per: Through, Fumes: Smoke)

- These are the substances made from natural or synthetic materials and are used for creating a pleasant odour.
- Perfumes are used to improve personal appearance in the society.
- They are used in cosmetics and in toilet preparations.
- The low quality perfumes are known as industrial odourants.
- Perfumes are mainly composed of volatile oils.
- Perfumes derived from plants are the volatile oils, also called as essential oils.
- Perfumes obtained from animal source are long lasting, hence are called as fixatives.

Examples

- *Flowers*: Rose, jasmine.
- *Stem*: Sandal.
- *Leaves*: Citronella.
- *Aerial parts*: Geranium.

Flavouring Agents

- These are the agents used to give a pleasant flavour to the formulations.
    i. Flavouring agents improve psychological effect of the preparations.
    ii. They are used to cover unpleasant odour and taste of the preparations.
    iii. Flavouring agents should be selected carefully.
    iv. It should not interact with substances present in the preparations.
    v. They should be capable of covering unpleasant odour and taste, e.g.
        - *To cover acidic taste*: Orange and liquorice.
        - *To cover bitter taste*: Fennel and peppermint.
        - *To cover salty taste*: Lemon and orange.
    vi. The flavours used from natural sources are lemon, mint, orange, clove, lavendor, rose, etc.

Q 18. Explain the following chemical tests:

a. Kellar-Killiani test (S. 98, 99, 00, 02, 07, 09; W. 98, 99, 03)
b. Borntrager test (S. 05, 06, 09)

a. Keller-Killiani Test for Digitoxose (for Cardiac Glycosides)

- 1 gm of powdered digitalis + 10 ml of 70% alcohol.
- Boil for 2–3 minutes and filter.
- Filtrate + 5 ml water + 0.5 ml lead acetate solution.
- Shake well and filter.
- Filtrate + equal volume of chloroform.
- Evaproate.
- Residue + acetic acid + 2 drops of $FeCl_3$.
- Transfer the mixture into test tube containing 2 ml of concentration H_2SO_4.

Observation

Reddish brown layer becomes bluish green in colour.

Conclusion

Digitoxose is present (cardiac glycoside).

b. Borntrager Test for Senna (Anthraquinone Glycosides) (S. 96, 98, 99, 01, 07, W. 96, 99, 02)

- Powdered leaves of senna + dilute HCl.
- Boil and filter immediately.
- Cool the filtrate.
- Filtrate + chloroform.
- Shake well and separate organic solvent layer.
- Add dilute ammonia to layer of organic solvent.

Observation

Ammoniacal layer becomes pink and finally red.

Conclusion

Anthraquinone glycosides are present.

Q 19. Give the difference between 'hydrolysable tannins' and 'condensed tannins'. (S. 09; W. 06)

Hydrolysable tannins	Condensed tannins
1. They undergo hydrolysis with the help of mineral acids like HCl, HNO_3, H_2SO_4	1. They cannot be hydrolysed. These are true tannins which on acid or enzyme treatment produce red insoluble compounds known as 'phlobaphenes'.
2. With ferric chloride solution they produce blue colour.	2. With ferric chloride solution they produce brownish green colour.
3. On dry distillation, gallic acid and other compounds gets converted into pyrogalol.	3. On dry distillation, they yield catechol tannin.
4. These are of two types: Galli tannins and ellagi tannins.	4. These are not classified further.
5. Examples: Rhubarb, clove, behda, myrobalan.	5. Examples: Catechu, cinchona.

Q 20. Describe general method of collection of bark. (W. 01)

Barks are collected in a season when they contain maximum concentration and active constituent. Following are methods of collecting barks:

a. Felling Method

This is very old method of collecting barks. The tree is cut at base and bark is peeled out.

b. Uprooting Method

In this method, roots of the plants are drawn out of soil and bark is stripped off from roots and branches.

c. Coppicing Method

In this method, plant is allowed to grow for a definite period and then it is cut off at specific distance from soil. The stumps, which remain in ground are allowed to send shoots, which develop further independently yielding aerial parts.

These new parts are cut off and bark is collected from shoots.

Q 21. Define and classify terpenoids with examples. (S. 04, 08)

Terpenoids are the hydrocarbons and their originated derivatives which are found in all volatile oils of plant or animal origin.

Classification of Terpenoids

Terpenoids are classified on the basis of isoprene units, i.e. C_5H_8.
1. Monoterpenes, e.g. camphor, tulsi, dill, coriander.
2. Sesquiterpenes, e.g. clove, sandalwood oil.
3. Diterpenoids, e.g. taxus.
4. Tritepenoids, e.g. ambergris.
5. Tetraterpenoids, e.g. annatto, crocus.
6. Polyterpenoids, e.g. rubber.

Q 22. State different techniques/methods of isolation of volatile oils. (S. 06. 07; W. 08)

1. Hydrodistillation

Method comprising of water distillation, water and steam distillation is used for extraction of volatile oil from herbal drugs. The fresh material is subjected to hydrodistillation in case of the leafy drug.

2. Enfleurage

This method is used for extraction of delicate perfumes. The fresh flower petals are mechanically spread on layer of fatty material, allowed to imbibe and exhausted petals are replaced by fresh material. The process is continued till fatty layer is saturated with volatile principles which are then extracted with lipid solvent.

3. Eucelle Method

This method is used for extraction of citrus oil, where in oil cells in ring are reptured mechanically using pointed projection by twisting raw material over them in clockwise direction either mechanically or mannually.

Q 23. What are glycosides? How are they isolated from plant? (W. 07)

Glycosides

Glycosides are defined as organic compounds from plant or animal sources which on enzymatic or acid hydrolysis gives one or more sugar moeities along with nonsugar moeities.

Method of Isolation of Glycosides

Stass-Otto Method

The drug containing glycoside is finely powdered and the powder is extracted by continuous hot percolation using Soxhlet's apparatus with alcohol as solvent.

During this process, various enzymes present in plant parts are also deactivated due to heating. The thermolabile glycoside should be extracted at temperature below 45°C. The extract is treated with lead acetate to precipitate tannin and thus eliminate nonglycosidal impurities. The excess of lead acetate is precipitated as lead sulphide by passing hydrogen sulphide gas through solution. The extract is filtered, concentrated to get crude glycosides.

From the crude extract the glycosides are obtained in pure form by making use of processes like crystallization, chromatographic techniques, etc.

Q 24. Describe the general method of isolation of tannins.

Isolation of Tannins

Both hydrolysable and condensed tannins are highly soluble in water and alcohol but insoluble in organic solvents like solvent ether, chloroform and benzene.

Tannin compounds can be easily extracted by water or alcohol. The general method for the extraction by water or alcohol. The general method for the extraction of tannic acid from various galls is either with water saturated ether or with mixture of water alcohol and ether. In such cases the free acids like gallic and ellagic acid goes along with ether while true tannins gets extracted in water. If drug consists of chlorophyll or pigment, may be removed by ether. After extraction the aqueous and etheral layers are separated concentrated, dried and subjected to further isolation and purification using various separational techniques of chromatography.

CHAPTER 6

Surgical Fibres, Sutures and Dressings

Q 1. What are fibres? Classify surgical fibres with examples. (S. 98, 07, 09; W. 00, 01)

Fibres

Fibres are the elements which are synthesized or prepared from plant or animal and contains chain of molecules.

Classification of Fibres

- Plant fibres, e.g. cotton, banana, jute.
- Animal fibres, e.g. silk, wool.
- Mineral fibres, e.g. glass, asbestos.
- Synthetic fibres, e.g. rayon, nylon, terylene.

Q 2. Define surgical dressings? Give its essential requirements. Mention uses of surgical dressings. (S. 04, W. 07)

Surgical Dressings

"The surgical dressings are the materials used for covering the wounds or injuries and to be applied singly or in combination."

Official/Essential Requirements

- They should be sterile.
- They should be stored in dry well-ventilated place at temperature not exceeding 25°C.
- There should not by any loose fibre.
- Adhesive products should not be allowed to freeze.
- Only permitted antiseptics should be used in a prescribed concentration.
- They should be dyed if mentioned in the monograph.

Uses of Surgical Dressings/Functions

- They provide ideal conditions for wound healing.
- They remove wound exudates from the site.
- They gives mechanical support to the tissues.
- They gives protection to healing wound.
- They prevents infections.
- They protects the wounds from outside liquids.

Q 3. What are different types of surgical dressings (classification). (S. 98, 00, 01; W. 96)

Types of Surgical Dressings

- Fibres and related materials, e.g. wood cellulose.
- Carded products, e.g. absorbent cotton.
- Nonextensible, nonadhesive woven products, e.g. absorbent muslin cloth.
- Nonextensible adhesible woven products, e.g. belladona adhesive plasters.
- Extensible nonadhesive products, e.g. cotton bandage, elastic web bandage.
- Extensible adhesive woven products, e.g. elastic adhesive bandage, extension plaster.
- Nonwoven products, e.g. surgical adhesive tape.

Q 4. What are sutures? What are the properties of sutures? Give uses. (S. 06; W. 99, 02)

Sutures

Sutures are sterile threads or fibres used for stiching or sewing the tissues together.

Properties of Sutures

- They must be sterile.
- They should be nonirritant.
- They should have finest possible gauge.
- They should have adequate strength.
- If absorbable, their time of absorption must be known.
- They are to be used once only.

Uses of Sutures

- Sutures are used for sewing the tissues together.

- Nylon sutures are used in skin and plastic surgery.
- Kangaroo tendons are speically used in hernia.
- Metallic sutures are used in general surgery.

Q 5. Define surgical sutures. How are they classified?

Surgical Sutures

"Surgical sutures are sterile threads or fibres used for stiching or sewing the tissues together."

Classification of Sutures

- Absorbable sutures:
  - i. Sterile catgut
  - ii. Sterile reconstituted collagen suture.
- Nonabsorbable sutures:
  - i. Fibres, e.g. silk, cotton
  - ii. Sterile linen suture, e.g. muslin
  - iii. Sterile polyamide suture, e.g. nylon
  - iv. Sterile polyester suture, e.g. terylene
  - v. Sterile stainless and silver suture, e.g. metal springs.
- Haemostatic sutures:
  - i. Oxidised cellulose
  - ii. Absorbable gelatin sponge.

Q 6. What is surgical catgut? Give the method of preparation of catgut.

Surgical Catguts

"Surgical catguts are the sterile absorbable sutures made of fibres obtained from collagen of animals."

Preparation of Catgut

- Collagen is obtained from submucus connective tissues of small intestine of sheep.
- Intestine is cleaned of its contents.
- About 7.5 meters of intestine is selected.
- It is split length wise in 2 to 3 ribbons.
- Ribbons are separated by machines.
- Ribbons are stretched under tension and dried. It gives mechanical strength to the ribbons.

- Ribbons are tanned or hardened by soaking them in a solution of chromium salt.
- The dried ribbons are polished to obtain smooth string gauzed for its diameters.
- The fine fibres having uniform diameters and smoothness are then sterilized.

Q 7. How catguts/sutures are sterilized? (S. 96, 97, 00; W, 97, 99)

The sterilization of catgut is done by following methods:

- *Chemical sterilization/iodine method*: In this method catguts are deeped in iodine and potassium iodide solution for 24 hours.
- *Sterilisation by irradiation*: This is the latest method. The catguts are exposed to gamma rays obtained from cobalt 60.
- *Sterilization by heat*: There are two methods:
  i. *Boilable catguts:* The catguts are placed in glass tube and are filled with some amount of Toulene and are heated. Then they are sterilized in autoclave. They are stored as a soaking material in distilled water.
  ii. *Nonboilable catguts*: The catguts are packed in plastic packets. They are placed in mixture of alcohol and water.

Q 8. Define the terms 'ligatures' and 'catguts'.

Ligatures

Ligatures are sterile threads or fibres used for tightening muscles, blood vessels, etc.

Bandage

A material which holds the dressing in place and applies pressure or support on injured parts is called bandage.

Q 9. Differentiate between surgical dressing and suture. (S. 99, 02; W. 98)

Surgical dressing	Suture
i. These includes all materials either used alone or along with others to cover the wounds.	i. These are sterile thread strings specially prepared for use in surgery for sewing tissues together.

Contd.

Surgical Dressing	Suture
ii. Function of surgical dressing is to protect the wounds and promote wound healing.	ii. Function is for sewing or stiching tissues.
iii. Surgical dressings have to comply certain properties, e.g. sterility, should not have loose fibres and ends in dressing.	iii. Sutures have to comply with certain properties, e.g. Non-irritation, adequate strength, sterility.
iv. Examples: Absorbent cotton, bandage.	iv. Examples: Oxidised cellulose, nylon, muslin.

Q 10. Give the biological source, method of preparation and uses of cotton. (S. 96, 98, 00, 01, 05, 06, 09; W. 98, 99, 02, 04, 08)

Cotton

- *Synonyme*: Absorbent cotton, cotton wool, purified cotton, gossypol.
- *Biological source*: The drug is obtained from trichomes of seeds of "Gossypium barbadense".
- *Family*: Malvaceae.

Method of Preparation of Absorbent Cotton

- The cotton plant after flowering bears the fruits known as capsules.
- Each capsule is made up of 3 to 5 chambers known as cells/seeds.
- They are covered by large number of trichomes.
- Each seed covered with trichomes is known as balls.
- After collecting the balls, they are subjected to ginning process.
- In ginning process, trichomes are separated from seeds.
- These trichomes with some instrument are divided into two types depending upon the length, as short fibres and long fibres.
- The short fibres are used in surgical dressings. They are known as linters.
- The raw cotton contains wax, fats, colouring matter and iron impurities.
- To remove the impurities, the linters are taken to "cotton opener".
- The fibres are then treated with dilute NaOH solution under pressure for 10 to 15 hours. It separates wax and fat from fibres.
- The fibres are washed with water, bleached, dried and sterilized.

Storage

- To be stored in cool and dry place.
- They should be protected from light.

Uses

- As a surgical dressings as ligature and suture.
- As a filter media.
- As insulator.
- It absorbs, blood, mucus, pus and prevents the wounds from infection.

Q 11. Write in brief about "wool". (W. 03)

Wool

- *Biological source*: They are obtained from the fleece of sheep ovis aries.
- *Family*: Bovidae.
- *Preparation*: The fleece of a sheep is cut and hairs are separated. Impurities like dust, grease are removed. The fibres are bleached, washed, dried sterilized and marketed.
- *Description*: Wool hairs are smooth, elastic, lustorus, curly, hygroscopic and slippery to touch.
- *Chemical constituents*: Keratin and cystine (amino acid).
- *Uses*:
    - i. Surgical dressing as ligature and sutures.
    - ii. Filter medium.
    - iii. In crape bandages.

Q 12. Give the biological source, method of preparations and uses of "silk". (S. 04, 07, 08; W. 01, 06, 07)

Silk

- *Biological source*: They are obtained from *cocoons* of *Bombyx mori* and other varities of Bombyx.
- *Family*: Bombycidae.

Method of Preparation

- In the life cycle of silk worm larva is the main stage.
- The larvae have some special glands in oral cavities.
- They secretes the fibre known as sericin, which on exposure to air becomes hard and form the cocoon.

- The cocoons are collected and heated at a temperature 60° to 80°C in steam current.
- The cocoon get opened.
- They are placed in hot water to dissolve the gum like substances and fibres becomes soft.
- The fibres are separated, sterilised, packed and marketed.
- *Chemical constituents*: Silk contain a protein known as fibroin.
- *Uses*:
    i. In surgical dressings as a ligature and suture.
   ii. In manufacturing of sieves.
  iii. In textiles.

CHAPTER 7

Adulteration, Drug Evaluation and Significance of Pharmacopoeial Standards

Q 1. What is adulteration? What are different methods of adulteration? (S. 99, 00, 01, 04, 07, 08, 09; W. 96, 98, 01, 02, 03, 04, 06, 07, 08)

Adulteration

"It is defined as worthless admixture of any material in the genuine drug."

Methods of Adulteration

• Mixing of materials obtained from same source, e.g. Bark can be adulterated by addition of stem pieces, cloves are mixed with cloves talks.

• Mixing of closely related parts of plants, e.g. leaves are supposed to be adulterated if the sample contains excessive amount of petioles.

• Mixing of exhausted drugs: The containing volatile oils are commonly adulterated in this way, e.g. exhausted fennel is added to genuine fennel.

• Roots and rhizomes are supposed to be adulterated if soil attached is not removed completely, e.g. ginger, gention have adulteration of soil attached with them.

• Mixing of natural substances appearing same as drugs, e.g. oils.

• Mixing of materials by making them similar to drug, e.g. tea granules can be adulterated by mud and tea powder by soil.

• Mixing of same part of the plant of different varieties, e.g. senna leaflet with arabic senna, dog senna. Ginger with African ginger, Japanese ginger.

• Adulteration to fortified inferior natural drugs, e.g. lemon grass oil can be adulterated by adding higher amount of citral.

- Substitution by artificially manufactured substitutes: This is observed in case of drugs which are costly, e.g. artificial invert sugar is mixed with honey.
- Many a times a synthetic chemical which constitutes one of the chemical constituents of the drug is added to the genuine drugs, e.g. benzyl benzoate to balsam of Peru and citral to oil of lemon grass and camphor oil and eucalyptus oil in oil of rose mary.

Q 2. Define drug evaluation. Give objective/importance of drug evaluation. (S. 99, 01, 03; W. 96, 97, 98, 99, 01, 07)

Definition

Evaluation of drug means confirmation of identity purity and quality of drugs.

Objectives of Drug Evaluation

- Confirmation of already existing standards as per pharmacopoeia.
- Detection of adulteration and substitution in the drug.
- To study variations in biochemical activities of drugs.
- To study deterioration of the drug due to storage of any chemical reaction.

Q 3. Enlist different methods of drug evaluation. (S. 97, 01, 03, 08; W. 97, 98, 99, 00)

- Morphological/organoleptic method.
- Microscopical method.
- Physical method.
- Chemical method.
- Biological method.

Q 4. Write a note on morphological/organoleptic method of drug evaluation. (S. 98, 01, 05, 09; W. 96, 98, 00, 01, 03, 04, 08)

- In this method morphological characters of the drugs are studied.
- This method is also known as organoleptic method because observations are taken with sensory organs.
- It is also known as macroscopical method because in the method generally entire drugs are examined.
- In this method following morphological characters are studied.
    i. Shape: Parts of the plants such as leaves, roots, barks, flowers have specific shape. Thus change is shape can be found and useful for evaluation.

ii. Colour: The colour of the drug dependant upon state of maturity of entire plant as well as cells of specific part. Thus colour change due to storage may be find out, e.g. Beeswax in crude state is yellowish-brown and when purified and bleached appears a white in colour.

iii. Odour: It is the observation taken with nose.

It plays an important role in identifying unorganised drugs and oils, e.g.

Aromatic odour: Fennel, coriander

Pungent: Clove

Pleasant: Peppermint.

iv. Taste: It is the observation taken with tongue. It is useful to identify unorganised drugs and oils, e.g. sweet—liquorice, bitter—nux vomica, sour and acrid—amla.

v. Fracture: It means broken surface of the bark. The drugs are broken with hands and broken surface is observed for the type of fracture, e.g. short fracture, granular fracture, fibrous fracture, sphintary fracture, laminated fractures.

vi. Part of plant: The various parts of plant are roots, stem, leaves, flowers, fruits, seeds, bulbs, leaflets, etc. Thus by knowing the part of plant in the sample, one can get an idea about the name of drug, e.g. root—Rauwolfia, leaf—Senna, Vasaka, Flower bud—Clove.

Merits/Advantages of Morphological Method

- Easy method.
- It helps in identification of drug.
- No special equipment is required.
- No special experimentation is required.
- It helps in deciding purity of drug.

Demerits/Disadvantages of Morphological Method

- Large quantity of sample is required during evaluation.
- Limitation of sensory organs of human being.
- Chances of sample to sample variation are observed.
- Applicable to entire organised crude drug.
- Time consuming method.
- Less helpful for unorganised drugs, powdered drugs and liquid drugs.

Q 5. Write a note on "microscopical evaluation" of crude drugs. (S. 00, 01, 02, 07, 08; W. 05)

- In this method observations are taken by using microscope.
- The microscopical characters of crude drugs such as trichomes. starch grains, stomata are observed under microscope.

Objectives of Microscopical Evaluation

- To study cellular arrangement in the drugs.
- To study special structures or tissues or any modifications.
- To take numerical measurements, e.g. number of stomata.
- To locate the site of various chemical constituents.

Types of Microscopical Evaluation

- *Qualitative microscopical method*: It helps in identification and to study cellular arrangement in the drug. In this method TS of drug is observed under microscope to observe Arenchyma, phloem, xylem, oil glands, stomata, trichomes, etc.
- *Quantitative microscopical method*: In this method numerical measurements are taken using microscope, e.g. number of starch grains, stomatal index, vein islet number. There is a fixed value or number for each and every standard of drug and it surely differs from its varieties, substituent and adulterants.
- *The Microchemical tests*: In this method chemical tests are performed on TS of drugs and they are observed for the presence or absence of chemical constituents. Under the microscope, e.g Agar powder + Ruthenium red → Red colour (mucilage is present).

Merits/Advantages

- Small quantity of sample is required.
- No person to person variation in observations.
- Standard observations and values are available in books.
- It can be applied to entire drug, powdered drug, rarely unorganised drug.
- It gives correct idea of substituents and adulterants.
- It confirms purity of drug.
- It helps in fixing location of constituents.

Demerits/Disadvantages

- Time consuming method.
- Skilled person is required for experimentation.

- Costly method.
- Does not give much more information about quality of drugs.
- Little application in unorganised drugs and oils.

Q 6. Write a note on "physical method of evaluation". (S. 09; W. 02)

In this method physical properties of drugs are studied. The experimental observations are compared with standard information. The variations in these two indicate pure nature of the sample. The following are physical properties of drugs useful in physical evaluation.

- *Viscosity*: Viscosity can be studied for oils and semiliquids. If the oil undergoes rancidity, condensation, the viscosity increases.
- *Density*: Adulterated oils have different densities than genuine oils.
- Optical activity: It helps in identifying the adulterants in the drug by considering changes in optical rotation.
- *Refractive index*: It is used in identification of volatile oils, fixed oils, fats, resins. The refractive index may changes as per temperature, pressure and light.
- *Melting point and boiling point*: Purity of drug is related to MP and BP. Hence BP and MP helps in identification and establishing purity of drugs.
- *Moisture content*: Estimation of moisture content is the estimation of H_2O content present in the drug. In case of moisture sensitive drugs definite moisture content is necessary. Hence it should be determined and controlled. The moisture control is necessary to prevent the destruction of crude drug due to chemical change or due to microbial contamination.
- *Ash value* (Ash content): Ash is a residue left after complete ignition of drug. It is expressed as % of ash collected on complete ignition of drug and compared with standard value to observe presence of impurity.
- *Extractive value*: The drug is extracted with organic solvents like water, alcohol, ether. Extractive values are important in identifying and determination of purity of drug.

Merits/Advantages of Physical Evaluation

- Useful for organised and unorganised drugs.
- Mainly applicable to unorganised, semisolids and liquids.

- Vegetative adulteration can be examined.
- Purity of drugs can be examined.
- Standard values of physical constants are available in official books.

Demerits/Disadvantages of Physical Evaluation

- Costly method.
- Time consuming method.
- The observation changes depending upon experimental conditions.
- It does not give information about quality of drugs.
- Skilled person is required to handle analytical equipment.

Q 7. Write a note on "chemical method" of drug evaluation. (S. 99, 04; W. 97, 99)

This method helps in determining chemical nature and chemical composition of drug.

- Objectives:
  i. Determination of active chemical constituents.
  ii. Determination of other chemical constituents.
  iii. Determination of % of active constituents.
  iv. Establishing quality of drug.
  v. Confirmation of variety of drug.
  vi. Confirmation of adulterant, if present.
- The chemical method involves three parts:
  i. *Solubility*: The solubility has more importance in the cases of unorganised drugs and oils. Solubility is important step in identification of drugs. The observations are noted in terms of freely soluble, soluble, sparingly soluble, insoluble, etc. For example, alkaloids and glycosides are soluble in alcohol. Carbohydrates and gums are completely soluble in water. Thus solubility helps in identification of drug and adulterant.
  ii. *Qualitative chemical test*: These are the simple chemical tests performed in order to identify various chemical constituents present in the drug. The drugs are powdered and treated with one or more reagents in a proper sequence and observations are noted, e.g. hydrolysable tannins gives blue colour with $FeCl_3$ solution and condensed tannins gives green/black colour with $FeCl_3$ solution.
  iii. *Quantitative chemical analysis method*: In this method % of active constituent is determined.

- *Assay*: The estimation of percentage purity of the active chemical constituent is known as assay.
- The important types of chemical assay are:
  - i. Volumetric assay:
    - Acid-base titration
    - Redox titration
    - Complexometric titration
    - Precipitation titration.
  - ii. Gravimetric assay.
  - iii. Potentiometric assay.
  - iv. Colourimetric assay.

Merits/Advantages of Chemical Method

- The experiments have a great accuracy.
- No chances of personal variation.
- Presence of chemical constituents in amounts can be determined.
- Confirmation to variety of drugs and adulterants present can be obtained.
- It determines the quality and purity of drugs
- It helps in judging pharmacological actions of the drugs.
- This method gives guidelines for extraction of crude drugs with the help of solubility.

Demerits/Disadvantages of Chemical Method

- Requires heavy instrumentation, so costly method.
- Skilled persons are required for experimental work.
- The pharmacological action predictable should be confirmed by using biological method.

Q 8. Write a note on "biological method" of evaluation. (S. 03; W. 06)

In this method the experimentation is carried on biological system, i.e. living organisms.
- Objectives
  - i. To study quantitative action of drugs.
  - ii. To study toxic effects of drugs.
  - iii. To study synergistic effects or antagonist effects of drugs.

Depending upon experimental animals biological methods can be divided as follows:

i. *Bioassay*: The estimation of potency of active constituent of crude drugs by means of its effect on living organisms is called as bioassay.

The bioassay can be studied using experimental animals or isolated tissues, e.g. heart and blood vessels—frog, eye—rabbit, respiration—dog.

The drugs are administered in the above animals in a particular dilutions with specific doses and the quantitative effects are observed.

ii. *Bacteriological assay method*: In this method the drug is evaluated by taking the actions of drugs on the growth of bacteria.

In this method a pure strain of microorganisms is introduced in nutrient medium and system is incubated at 37°C for sufficient length of time.

A series of solution of various dilutions are prepared. The selected dilutions are administered in the nutrient medium in a definite doses.

The system is again incubated and effects are noted.

Merits/Advantages Biological Method of Evaluation

- It helps in determination of potency of drug.
- It also helps in determination of ED_{50} and LD_{50}.
- Effect on various systems can be studied.
- It gives idea about quality of drugs.
- Synergistic agents and antagonists can be find out.
- Toxic effects of drug can be find out.
- Used when other methods of evaluation cannot be used.

Demerits/Disadvantages Biological Method of Evaluation

- Very complicated method.
- Costly method.
- Time consuming method.
- Skilled person is required for experimentation.
- Does not given an idea about morphological, physical or chemical properties of drugs.
- Animals are required for experimentation.

Q 9. Give difference between "leaf and leaflet" and "oil and fat". (S. 05)

Leaf	Leaflet
i. In case of leaves, bud or branch is present in the axil.	i. It is absent in leaflets.
ii. Leaves are arranged spirally.	ii. Leaflets are arranged in pairs.
iii. Leaves lie in different planes.	iii. Leaflets lie in the same plane.
iv. Leaves are generally symmetrical at the base.	iv. Leaflets are asymmetrical at the bases.
v. Examples: Digitalis, vasaka.	v. Examples: Senna, neem, rose.

Oil	Fat
i. These are substances which remain liquid at 15–16°C.	i. These are the substances which remain solid at 15–16°C.
ii. They contains less amount of saturated acids.	ii. They contain more % of saturated acids.
iii. Oils can be subclassified as drying oils, semidrying oils and nondrying oils.	iii. Fats cannot be subclassified.
iv. Examples: Linseed oil, castor oil, amond oil.	iv. Examples: Coconut oil, cocoa butter.

Q 10. How moisture content is useful in evaluation of drugs? (W. 07)

- Moisture content means amount of water content present in the drug.
- Water is essential component of living organisms but some drugs a less stable in water.
- In case of the moisture sensitive drugs, definite moisture is necessary.
- The moisture control is necessary to prevent the destruction of crude drugs either due to chemical change or due to microbial contamination.
- Excessive presence of water may lead into fungal and microbial growth, affecting chemical nature of drug, stability and pharmacological action.

- Moisture content can be determined by:
  - i. Heating the drug in an oven at 100°C until the weight is constant.
  - ii. Karl Fisher reagent is used to determine moisture content.

Q 11. Explain "ash value" (ash content). (W. 08)

- Ash is a residue after complete ignition of the drug.
- In experiment a carefully weighed quantity of a drug is taken into porcelain crucible and it is burned completely.
- Ash collected is heated at 450°C to remove organic content of drug.
- Heating is continued till two constant weight of the ash are obtained then the percentage of change in weight is calculated.
- Importance of ash value:
  - i. It helps in identification of drugs.
  - ii. It helps in deciding purity of drug.
  - iii. It helps in detecting the adulteration and substitutions.
- Acid insoluble ash: It is the % of ash which is insoluble in dilute HCl.
- Water soluble ash: When above observation fails, the ash is treated with water and % of water soluble ash is calculated.

Q 12. How "extractive values" are helpful in drug evaluation? (S. 96)

Extraction of drug is done with solvents such as water, alcohol, ether. Extractive values are important in identification of drugs and determination of purity of drugs.

  i. *Water soluble extractive value*: The drugs containing carbohydrates, plant acids, tannins are tested for their solubility in water.

  ii. *Alcohol soluble extractive value*: The drugs containing alkaloids, resins, glycosides are tested for their solubility in 90% alcohol.

  iii. *Ether soluble extractive value*: It is important for the drugs containing volatile oils, fixed oils and colouring matter.

Q 13. Define bark. What are various shapes/types of barks?

Bark

Barks are the external tissues of stems.

Types of Barks

1. *Flat barks:* The barks are collected from large plants and shows flat surface, e.g. Arjuna bark.

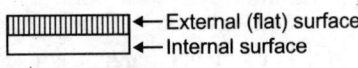

2. *Curved barks:* The barks are collected from primary branches of stems, e.g. Ashoka.

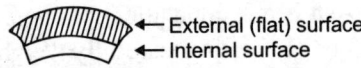

3. *Recurved barks:* The barks are collected from primary branches containing the more soft tissues. The shape can be explained as concavity on the external surface , e.g. Kurchi.

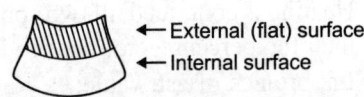

4. *Channeled barks:* The barks are collected from secondary branches of the stem. The curvature is more but the ends are not meeting each others, e.g. Cascara.

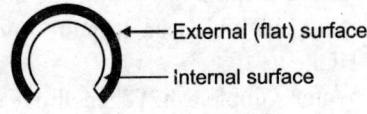

5. *Double quilled barks:* Two ends of bark are quilled, e.g. cascara in rare cases.

6. *Compound quilled barks:* One quill is inserted in other quilled, e.g. Cinnamon.

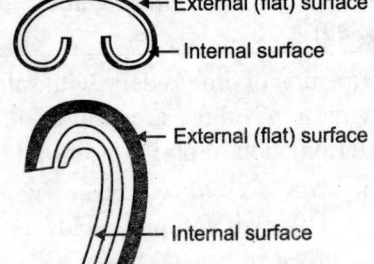

Q 14. Define fractures. Explain various types of fractures?

Fractures

Fractures are the transverse broken surfaces of the bark.

Types of Fractures

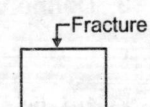

1. *Short fracture:* The surface is smooth, e.g. Kurchi bark.

2. *Granular fracture:* The surface shows small circular elevations, e.g. wild cherry bark.

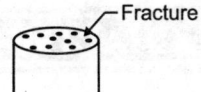

3. *Fibrous fracture:* Fibre like materials project out on breaking the drug, e.g. cinchona, ginger.

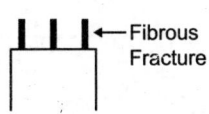

4. *Sphintary fracture:* The surface shows various levels or steps, e.g. Cinnamon bark.

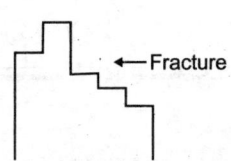

5. *Laminated fracture:* The drug cannot be broken in single plane, e.g. Quassia root.

CHAPTER 8

Pharmacological Grouping of Natural Drugs

A LAXATIVES

Q 1. Define the term laxatives. Name the four drugs used as laxative. (S. 96, 00, 01, 03, 06, 07, 09; W. 99, 08)

- *Laxatives*: The drugs which promotes defaecation are called laxatives.
- *Drugs*: Aloe, senna, castor oil, rhubarb, ispaghula.
- *Laxatives*: These are categoriesed as:
  - i. *Laxatives*: It means elimination of soft formed stools, e.g. senna, isapgol, liquid-paraffin.
  - ii. *Purgatives*: It means more evacuation of stools, e.g. castor oil, aloe, rhubarb.
  - iii. *Drastics*: They act intensely by irritating the mucous membrane of the intestine, e.g. jalap, podophyllum.
  - iv. *Hydrogogue*: It means the substances which produce fluid motions, e.g. cotton oil, colocynth.

Q 2. Give the synonyms, biological source, chemical constituents and uses of the following crude drugs: a. Senna, b. Aloe, c. Castor oil, d. Rhubarb, e. Ispaghula.

a. Senna (S. 99, 01, 02, 03; W. 07)

- *Synonyms*: Sonamukhi, Tinevelly senna, Indian senna.
- *Biological source*: It consists of dried leaflets of cassia angustifolia vahl.
- *Family*: Leguminosae.
- *Chemical constituents*: Senna contains anthraquinone glycosides.
  - i. Sennoside A

    ii. Sennoside B

    iii. Sennoside C

    iv. Sennoside D

    v. Sennidin

    vi. Rhein

    vii. Emodin

    viii. Aloe-emodin.

- *Uses*: Senna leaves are used as laxatives.
- *Substitutes and adulterants*:
  i. Dog senna
  ii. Arabian senna.

b. Aloe (S. 99,00, 02, 03; W. 01, 03)

- *Synonyms*: Korphad, musabbar, kumari.
- *Biological source*: Aloe is the dried juice of the leaves of Aloe *barbadensis* miller.
- *Family*: Liliaceae.
- *Chemical constituents*:
  i. Aloin
  ii. Barbaloin
  iii. Isobarbaloin
  iv. Aloe-emodin
  v. β-barbaloin
  vi. Resin contain aloesin.
- *Uses*:
  i. Aloe is used as purgative.
  ii. Used in cosmetics as protective.
  iii. Stimulates the growth of hairs.
  iv. Also applied for painful inflammations.

c. Castor oil (S. 96; W. 97, 01)

- *Synonyms*: *Oleum ricini*, ricinus oil.
- *Biological source*: Castol oil is a fixed oil obtained by the cold expression of the seeds of *Ricinus communis*.
- *Family*: Euphorbiaceae.
- *Chemical constituents*:
  i. Ricinoleic acid
  ii. Isoricinoleic acid

    iii. Linoleic acid
    iv. Isostearic acid
    v. Stearic acid.

- *Uses*:
    i. Castor oil is used as a cathartic.
    ii. As lubricant.
    iii. Used in preparations of paints, enamel, varnishes, greasy, polishes, printing ink.
    iv. Used in cosmetics.

d. Rhubarb

- *Synonyms*: Radix, rhein, rheum
- *Biological source*: Rhubarb consist of dried rhizome of rhein emodi wall.
- *Family*: Polygonaceae.
- *Chemical constituents*:
    i. Rhein
    ii. Emodin
    iii. Chrysophanol
    iv. Glucorhein
    v. Palmidin A, B, C
- *Uses*:
    i. Bitter stomachic   ii. Purgative

e. Ispaghula

- *Synonyms*: *P. psyllium*, Isabgol, Plantago.
- *Biological source*: Flowers of *Plantago ovata* and *P. arenaria*, *P. indicia*.
- *Zenus*
- *Chemical constituents*: Mucilage contains natural dietary fibre.
- *Uses*: The husk of the seeds is useful in constipation, cholesterol reduction and glycemic response. It is used in as a high fibre breakfast cereal.

B CARDIOTONICS

Q 3. Define cardiotonics. Give four examples. (S. 06, 07; W. 07)

- *Cardiotonics*: The drugs which increases the force of contraction of cardiac muscles and stimulates the overall activity of heart are called as cadiotonics, e.g. digitalis, strophanthus, squill, Arjuna bark.

Q 4. Give the synonyms, biological source, chemical constituents and uses of: a. Digitalis, b. Arjuna.

a. Digitalis (S. 96, 99, 00, 04, 05, 06, 07, 08; W. 03, 07)

- *Synonyms*: Fox glove leaves, digitalis leaves.
- *Biological source*: Digitalis consists of dried leaves of digitalis purpurea dried at a temperature below 60°C, immediately after collecting the leaves.
- *Family*: Scrophulariaceae.
- *Chemical constituents*: Digitalis contains cardiac glycosides:
    - i. Digoxin
    - ii. Digitoxin
    - iii. Gitoxin
    - iv. Digitoxigenin
    - v. Digitonin
    - vi. Gitonin
    - vii. Digoxigenin
    - viii. Purpurea glycosides A and B.
- *Uses*:
    - i. It is used as a cardiotonic
    - ii. In the treatment of congestive heart failure.

b. Arjuna

- *Synonyms*: Arjuna bark.
- *Biological source*: Arjuna consists of dried stem bark of the plant known as Terminatia Arjuna Rob.
- *Family*: Combretaceae.
- *Chemical constituents*:
    - i. Tannins (15%)
    - ii. Arjunolic acid
    - iii. Saponin
    - iv. Ellagic acid
    - v. Arjunic acid.
- *Uses of Arjuna*:
    - i. Used as a cardiotonic
    - ii. It is also used as a styptic and antidysenteric
    - iii. Arjuna bark is used extensively in tanneries and also as timber.

C CARMINATIVES AND GASTROINTESTINAL REGULATORS

Q 5. What are carminatives and GIT regulators? Give examples. (S. 97, 06, 07; W. 00, 01, 02)

- *Carminatives*: The drugs which expel the flatulence and gas from the gastrointestinal tract are called as carminatives, e.g. fennel, coriander, cardamom, clove, cinnamon, caraway.
- *Gastrointestinal regulators*: The drugs which regularise the activity of gastrointestinal tract are called as GI regulators, e.g. fennel, coriander, cinnamon, Caraway.

The gastrointestinal regulators includes stomachics, stimulants, aromatics, sialogogue, cholagogues, antiemetics, appetizers.

Q 6. Give the synonyms, biological source, chemical constituents and uses of following crude drugs: a. Ginger, b. Fennel, c. Coriander, d. Clove, e. Asafoetida, f. Nutmeg, g. Black pepper, h. Ajowan, i. Cinnamon.

a. Ginger (S. 96, 97, 04; W. 96, 97, 99, 01, 06)

- *Synonyms*: Gingerin, zingiber, zingiberis.
- *Biological source*: Ginger consists of rhizomes of *zingiber officinale.*
- *Family*: Zingiberaceae.
- *Chemical constituents*
    - i. Gingerol like shogaols, zingerone, gingediols
    - ii. Zingiberene
    - iii. Volatile oils (1–4%).
- *Uses*:
    - i. Stomachic
    - ii. Carminative
    - iii. Stimulant
    - iv. Flavouring agents.

b. Fennel (S. 96, 99, 01, 03, 05, 06; W. 97, 01, 05)

- *Synonyms*: Saunf, *Fructus foeniculum*, Badishep.
- *Biological source*: Fennel consists of dried ripe fruits of the plant known as *Foeniculum vulgare.*
- *Family*: Umbelliferae.
- *Chemical constituents*:
    - i. Fenchone

    ii. Anethole

    iii. Phellandrene

    iv. Limonene

    v. Anisidic aldehyde.

- *Uses*:

    i. Carminative

    ii. Aromatic

    iii. Stimulant

    iv. Expectorant

    v. Flavouring agent.

c. Coriander (S. 96, 00, 01, 02; W. 97)

- *Synonyms*: Coriander fruits, Dhania.
- *Biological source*: It consists of the fully dried ripe fruits of the plant known as *Coriandrum sativum* linn.
- *Family*: Umbelliferae.
- *Chemical constituents*:

    i. Geraniol

    ii. Pinene

    iii. L-borneol

    iv. D-linalool (coriandrol)

    v. Coriandryl acetate.

- *Uses*:

    i. Aromatic

    ii. Carminative

    iii. Stimulant

    iv. Flavouring agents.

d. Clove (S. 97, 05, 09; W. 99, 00, 01, 02)

- *Synonyms*: Clove flower, Clove buds, Lavang, Laung, Caryophyllum.
- *Biological source*: It consists of dried flower buds of *Eugenia caryophyllus*.
- *Family*: Myrtaceae.
- *Chemical constituents*:

    i. Eugenol

    ii. Eugenol acetate

    iii. Coryophyllenes

    iv. Volatile oil (15 to 20%)

    v. Eugenin.

- *Uses*:
    i. Dental analgesic
    ii. Carminative
    iii. Stimulant
    iv. Flavouring agent
    v. Aromatic
    vi. Antiseptic
    vii. The oil is used in perfumery and also in manufacture of vanillin

e. **Asafoetida (S. 96, 99, 00; W. 96, 97, 99, 00, 01, 02)**
- *Synonyms*: Devils dung, Hing, Gum asafoetida.
- *Biological source*: Asafoetida is the oleo-gum resin obtained by making incision from living rhizomes and roots of *Ferula foetida*.
- *Family*: Umbelliferae.
- *Chemical constituents*:
    i. Ferulic acid
    ii. Umbelliferone
    iii. Resin (40 to 65%)
    iv. Gum (20 to 25%)
    v. Volatile oil (4 to 20%).
- *Uses*:
    i. Carminative
    ii. Nervine tonic
    iii. Flavouring agent
    iv. Intestinal antiseptic
    v. In veterinary medicine.

f. **Nutmeg (S. 98, 00, 03; W. 96, 01)**
- *Synonyms*: Banda soap, Jayphal, Myristica, Nux moschata.
- *Biological source*: Nutmeg consists of dried kernels of seeds of *Myristica fragrans*.
- *Family*: Myristicaceae.
- *Chemical constituents*:
    i. Myristicin
    ii. Elimicin
    iii. Saffrole
    iv. Myristic, palmitic, oleic, lauriec acids.

- *Uses*:
  - i. Aromatic
  - ii. Stimulant
  - iii. Carminative
  - iv. Flavouring agent
  - v. Used in soap industries
  - vi. In the treatment of rheumatism.

g. Black Pepper (S. 96)

- *Synonyms*: Kali mirri, Kali mirch.
- *Biological source*: It consists of dried unriped fruits of *piper nigrum*.
- *Family*: Piperaceae.
- *Chemical constituents*:
  - i. Piperine
  - ii. Volatile oil (1 to 2.5%)
  - iii. Resin (6%)
  - iv. Piperidine
  - v. Starch.
- *Uses*:
  - i. Aromatic
  - ii. Stimulant
  - iii. Stomachic
  - iv. Carminative
  - v. As a condiment
  - vi. Used as a spice due to pungent taste.

h. Ajowan

- *Synonyms*: Carum copticum hieren, Trachyspermum copticum.
- *Biological source*: Ajowan consists of dried ripe fruits of plant, Tachyspermum ammi.
- *Family*: Umbelliferae.
- *Chemical constituents*:
  - i. Volatile oil contains thymol (35 to 60%)
  - ii. P-cymene (50 to 55%)
  - iii. Terpinene
  - iv. Pinene
  - v. Dipentenes.

- *Uses*:
    - i. Antispasmodic
    - ii. Stimulant
    - iii. Carminative
    - iv. In the treatment of sore throat, bronchitis
    - v. Antiseptic, insecticide.

i. Cinnamon

- *Synonyms*: Dalchini or Darchini.
- *Biological source*: Bark of the plant *Cinnamomum zeylanicum*.
- *Family*: Lauraceae.
- *Chemical constituents*: Essential oils, coumarin.
- *Uses*: Used as a spice in cooking, home remedies.

D ASTRINGENTS

Q 7. What are astringents and give examples. (S. 96, 99, 06, 07, 08; W. 99, 00, 02, 03, 05, 07)

- *Astringents*: Astringents are the drugs, which cause precipitation of protein.
- They are capable of arresting haemorrhages and reducing secretions of mucous membranes of stomach.
- Astringents are used as styptic and antidiarrhoeal agents.
  Natural astringents may be of:
    - i. *Vegetable*: Tannic acid, Catechu.
    - ii. *Mineral*: Copper and zinc, e.g. Black catechu, Pale catechu.

Q 8. Give the synonyms, biological source, chemical constituents and uses of following crude drugs: a. Black catechu, b. Pale catechu.

a. Black Catechu (S. 98, 02, 04, 05, 06; W. 96, 07)

- *Synonyms*: Kattha, Khair
- *Biological source*: It consists of dried aqueous extracts of the prepared from heart wood of *Acacia catechu* wild.
- *Family*: Leguminosae.
- *Chemical constituents*:
    - i. It contains about 10% of acacatechin.
    - ii. Quercetin
    - iii. Gum

iv. Catechu red

v. Quercitrin.

- *Uses*:

   i. It is used as astringents

   ii. Used in cough and diarrhoea

   iii. It has cooling and digested property.

b. Pale Catechu (S. 03, 06)

- *Synonyms*: Gambier, Gambir.
- *Biological source*: It is dried aqueous extracts of leaves and young shoots of *Uncaria gambier.*
- *Family*: Rubiaceae.
- *Chemical constituents*:

   i. Catechin

   ii. Catechu tannic acid

   iii. Catechu red

   iv. Gambier fluorescein.

- *Uses*:

   i. In treatment of diarrhoea

   ii. Local astringent in form of lozenges

   iii. Mainly used in dying and tannic industries.

E DRUGS ACTING ON CENTRAL NERVOUS SYSTEM (CNS)

   i. CNS stimulants: The drugs which stimulates the brain and spinal cord are called as CNS stimulants, e.g. Nux vomica, Lobelia.

   ii. CNS depressants: The drugs which depress the activities of CNS are called as CNS depressants, e.g. opium, ashwaggandha, cannabis.

1. Opium (S. 99, 01, 02, 05)

- *Synonym:* Raw opium.
- *Biological source*: It is the dried latex obtained by incisions from unripe capsules of *Papaver somniferum* linn.
- *Family*: Papaveraceae.
- *Chemical constituents*:

   i. Narcotine

   ii. Papaverine

   iii. Morphine

   iv. Codeine

   v. Thebaine.

- *Uses*:
  - i. Narcotic analgesic
  - ii. Hypnotic and sedative
  - iii. Codeine is used as antitussive.

2. **Hyoscyamus**
- *Synonym*: Henbane.
- *Biological source*: It consists of dried leaves and flowering tops of hyoscyamus niger.
- *Family*: Solanaceae.
- *Chemical constituents*:
  - i. Hyoscyamine
  - ii. Atropine
  - iii. Hyoscine.
- *Uses*:
  - i. It relieves spasms of urinary tract.
  - ii. It is used as sedative
  - iii. As expectorant, antispasmodic, antiasthmatic.

3. **Belladonna**
- *Synonyms*: Belladonna leaf, deadly nightshade leaf.
- *Biological source*: It consists of dried leaves of *Atropa belladonna*.
- *Family*: Solanaceae.
- *Chemical constituents*:
  - i. Atropine
  - ii. Hyoscyamine
  - iii. Hyoscine
  - iv. Homatropine.
- *Uses*:
  - i. It is used as anticholinergic
  - ii. It is used as antidote in opium and chloral hydrate poisoning.

4. **Aconite (S. 03; W. 96)**
- *Synonyms*: Aconit root, Bachnag, Monkshood.
- *Biological source*: It is the dried root of *Aconitum nepellus*.
- *Family*: Ranunculaceae.
- *Chemical constituents*
  - i. Aconitine
  - ii. Hypacotinine

iii. Neoline

iv. Aconitic acid.

* *Uses*:

  i. Externally in the form of liniment in treatment of neuralgia, sciatica, rheumatism and inflammation.

  ii. It is also used as analgesic and cardiac depressant.

5. Ashwagandha (S. 98, 05, 08; W. 96, 01)

* *Synonyms*: Withania root, Asgandh.
* *Biological source*: It consists of dried roots and stem bases of *Withania somnifera*.
* *Family*: Solanaceae.
* *Chemical constituents*:

  i. Withanine

  ii. Withaferine

  iii. Withanolides.

* *Uses*:

  i. It has sedative and hypnotic effect.

  ii. It is hypotensive and respiratory stimulant.

  iii. It is used in the treatment of gout, rheumatism and hypertension.

6. Cannabis

* *Synonyms*: Cannabis indica, Indian hemp, ganja.
* *Biological source*: Cannabis consists of dried flowering tops of cultivated female part of *Cannabis sativa* linn.
* *Family*: Cannabinaceae.
* *Chemical constituents*:

  i. Cannabinol

  ii. Cannabigerol

  iii. Tetrahydro cannabinol

  iv. Cannabidiol.

* *Uses*: It is used as narcotic sedative and analgesic.

7. Ephedra (S. 98, 99, 05; W, 96, 97, 00, 05)

* *Synonym*: Ma huang.
* *Biological source*: It consist of dried young stems of *ephedra gerardina* wall.
* *Family*: Ephedraceae.

- *Chemical constituents*: It contains alkaloids such as:
  - i. Ephedrine
  - ii. Nor-ephedrine
  - iii. Pseudoephedrine.
- *Uses*:
  - i. As a bronchodilator in asthma.
  - ii. In treatment of allergic conditions like hay fever.

8. **Nuxvomica (S. 96, 97, 99, 02, 07; W. 96, 97, 98, 99, 00)**
- *Synonym*: Crow-fig.
- *Biological source*: It consists of dried ripe seeds of strychnos nux vomica linn.
- *Family*: Loganiaceae.
- *Chemical constituents*: It contains bitter indole alkaloids.
  - i. Strychnine
  - ii. Brucine
  - iii. Vomicine
  - iv. Pseudo-strychnine.
- *Uses*
  - i. As a bitter stomachic and tonic
  - ii. It is a CNS stimulant
  - iii. It increases blood pressure and recommended in certain forms of cardiac failure.

F ANTIHYPERTENSIVES

Q 9. What are antihypertensives and describe the drug rauwolfia. (S. 96, 01, 03, 07, 08; W. 97, 00, 01, 07)

Antihypertensives

Antihypertensives are the drugs, which lower elevated blood pressure to normal level, e.g. rauwolfia.

Rauwolfia

- *Synonyms*: Serpentine root, sarpagandha, chota chand.
- *Biological source*: Rauwolfia consists of dried roots of the plant known as rauwolfia serpentine Benth.
- *Family*: Apocyanaceae.
- *Chemical constituents*:
  - i. Reserpene is an important alkaloid
  - ii. Oleoresin

  iii. Phytosterol
  iv. Other alkaloids are ajmaline, ajmalicine, rauwolfinine, rescinnamine, reserpinine, serpentine, etc.
- *Uses*:
  i. Antihypertensive
  ii. To treat mild essential hypertension
  iii. It has tranquillizing effect used in mild anxiety conditions.
  iv. In the treatment of snake bite.

G ANTITUSSIVES

Q 10. What are antitussives? Give examples of antitussives. (S. 98, 99, 01, 02, 04, 05, 06, 07; W. 99, 00, 05)

Antitussives

Antitussives are the drugs used to assist in the removal of secretion or exudate from the trachea, bronchi or lungs and hence are useful in treatment of cough, e.g. Vasaka, Tolu Balsam, Tulsi.

Q 11. Give the synonyms, biological source, chemical constituents and uses of following crude drugs: a. Vasaka, b. Tolu Balsam, c. Tulsi.

a. Vasaka (S. 02, 05, 06, 07; W. 97)
- *Synonyms*: Adulsa, Adhatoda.
- *Biological source*: Vasaka consists of dried as well as fresh leaves of the plant Adhatoda vasica nees.
- *Family*: Acanthaceae.
- *Chemical constituents*:
  i. Vasicine
  ii. Vasicinone
  iii. 6-hydroxy vasicine
  iv. It contains volatile oil betain and vasakin.
- *Uses*:
  i. Expectorant ii. Bronchodilator.

b. Tolu Balsam
- *Synonym*: Balsam of tolu.
- *Biological source*: Balsam of tolu is solid or semisolid balsam obtained from the trunk of trees Myroxylon balsamum.

- *Family*: Leguminosae.
- *Chemical constituents*:
    - i. Cinnamic acid 8%
    - ii. Benzoic acid 7.6%
        - a. Benzyl benzoate
        - b. Benzyl cinnamate.
- *Uses*
    - i. Expectorant and flavouring agent
    - ii. Antiseptic
    - iii. Common ingredient in cough mixtures.

c. Tulsi (S. 00; W. 97, 99, 00, 01)

- *Synonyms*: Sacred basil, Holy basil.
- *Biological source*: Tulsi consists of fresh and dried leaves of Ocimum sanctum
- *Family*: Labiatae.
- *Chemical constituents*:
    - i. Eugenol 70%
    - ii. Carvacrol 3%
    - iii. Eugenol-methyl-ether 20%
    - iv. Fixed oil
    - v. It also contains traces of alkaloid, saponin, tannin, small amount of vitamin C, traces of maleic, oleic, tartaric acid.
- *Uses*:
    - i. Oil is used as antibacterial and insecticidal
    - ii. Leaves used as stimulant.

H ANTIRHEUMATICS

Q 12. What are antirheumatics and give examples of antirheumatics. (S. 01, 02, 07; W. 99, 03, 04)

Antirheumatics: The drugs used to relieve or used in treatment of rheumatism are known as antirheumatics.

Rheumatism is an inflammatory condition characterized by the macroglobulin known as RF in blood and synovial fluid, e.g. guggul, colchicum.

Q 13. Give the synonyms, biological source, chemical constituents and uses of following drugs: a. Guggul, b. Colchicum.

a. Guggul (S. 03)

- *Synonyms*: Scented bdellium, Gum guggul, Indian dellium.
- *Biological source*: Guggul is the oleo-resin obtained by the incision of the bark of plant Commiphora weightii.
- *Family*: Bruseraceae.
- *Chemical constituents*:
    - i. Steroids
    - ii. Diterpenoids
    - iii. Carbohydrates and aliphatic esters
    - iv. Myrecene
    - v. Caryophylline
    - vi. Z-guggulosterene
    - vii. E-guggulo-sterone.
- *Uses*
    - i. Anti-inflammatory
    - ii. Antirheumatic
    - iii. Hypolipedemic
    - iv. Hypocholesteremic.

b. Colchicum (S. 98, 01)

- *Synonyms*: Colchicum seeds.
- *Biological source*: Colchicum consists of dried seeds of the plant Colchicum luteum.
- *Family*: Liliaceae.
- *Chemical constituents*:
    - i. It contains 0.2 to 1% of colchicine
    - ii. Demecolcine
    - iii. Colchicoresin
    - iv. Starch.
- *Uses*:
    - i. Gout and rheumatism
    - ii. It controls the malignant tumour
    - iii. It is used to cause polyploidy
    - iv. Used in horticulture.

I ANTITUMOUR

Q 14. What are antitumour drugs and give example. (S. 96, 07; W. 98, 99)

Antitumour are the drugs used in treatment of tumour/cancer. Tumour is defined abnormal or uncontrolled cellular multiplication in neoplasm, e.g. vinca.

Q 15. Give synonyms, biological source, chemical constituents and uses of vinca.

Vinca (S. 98, 01, 07; W. 98, 02, 03)

*   *Synonyms*: Vinca rosea, catharanthus, periwinkle.
*   *Biological source*: It is dried whole plant of catharanthus roseus.
*   *Family*: Apocyanaceae.
*   *Chemical constituents*: It contains:
    i. 20 dimeric indole dihydroindole
    ii. Vincristine
    iii. Vinblastine
    iv. Ajmalicine
    v. Lochnerine
    vi. Serpentine
*   *Uses*:
    i. It is given in intravenously in treatment of acute leukemia
    ii. It is antineoplastic agent
    iii. In treatment of Hodgkin's disease
    iv. It suppresses immune response.

J ANTILEPROTICS

Q 16. What are antileprotics? Give example. (S. 98, 06, 07; W. 99)

Antileprotics are the drugs used in treatment of leprosy, e.g. Chaulmoogra oil.

Leprosy is an infectious disease caused by microorganism known as *Mycobacterium leprae*.

Q 17. Give synonyms, biological source, chemical constituents and uses of the following drugs.

Chaulmoogra Oil (S. 97, 00, 03, 07; W. 01, 04)

*   *Synonyms*: Hydnocarpus oil, Gynocardia oil.

- *Biological source*: It is the fixed oil obtained by cold expression method from ripe seeds of the plant Taraktogenos kurzii king.
- *Family*: Flacourtriaceae.
- *Chemical constituents*:
    - i. Chaulmoogric acid (27%)
    - ii. Hydnocarpic acid (48%)
    - iii. Glycerides of palmitic acid.
- *Uses*
    - i. It is used in tuberculosis
    - ii. Leprosy
    - iii. Psoriasis
    - iv. Rheumatism
    - v. It has bactericidal effect against *Mycobacterium leprae* and *Mycobacterium tuberculosis*.

K ANTIDIABETICS

Q 18. What are antidiabetics and give examples of antidiabetic drugs. (S. 06)

Antidiabetics are the drugs used to reduce elevated blood sugar level, e.g. a. pterocarpus b. Gymnema.

Q 19. Give synonyms, biological source, chemical constituents and uses of the following drugs.

a. Pterocarpus (S. 00, 02, 05; W. 99, 02)

- *Synonyms*: Bijasal, Indian kino tree, Malabar kino.
- *Biological source*: It consists of dried juice of plant *Pterocarpus marsupium* linn.
- *Family*: Leguminosae.
- *Chemical constituents*:
    - i. Kinotonnic acid 70–80% (glucosidal tannin)
    - ii. Kino red (it is anhydride of kionin)
    - iii. Catechol
    - iv. Gallic acid
- *Uses*
    - i. It is used as powerful astringent.
    - ii. In treatment of diarrhoea and dysentery.
    - iii. Used in dyeing, tanning and printing.
    - iv. Used in passive haemorrhage and toothache.

b. Gymnema (S. 01, 05; W. 02)
- *Synonyms*: Gudmar, Madhunashni.
- *Biological source*: It consists of leaves of perennial woody climber plant known as *Gymnema sylvestre*.
- *Family*: Asclepiadaoceae
- *Chemical constituents*: It contains:
    i. Pentriacontrane
    ii. Phytin
    iii. α and β chlorophylls
    iv. Gymnemic acid.
- *Uses*
    i. It is used as antidiabetic   iv. Laxative
    ii. Stamachic   v. Diuretic
    iii. Stimulant

L ANTIDYSENTERICS

Q 20. What are antidysenteric drugs? Give examples.

- *Antidysenteric drugs*: These are the drugs used in treatment of dysentery.

    The term dysentery is a combination of two words namely—dys means bad or difficult, enteron means intestine.

    In dysenteric conditions the inflammation of the colonic mucosa occurs which leads to passage of blood and mucus.

- Depending on the type of invading parasite, dysenteric condition is grouped in various types:
    i. *Anaerobic dysentery*: It occurs due to *Entamoeba histolytica* which infects the large intestine. Parasite invades the mucosa and causes ulcers. It occurs either in acute and chronic form.
    ii. *Bacillary dysentery*: It occurs due to various forms of dysentery bacilli viz. *Shigella*. These parasites attack the mucous membrane of large intestine causes necrosis.
        – It is severe than the amoebic dysentery.
    iii. *Balantidal dysentery*: In this type dysentery and diarrhoea are associated with presence of a large ciliate protozoan called *Balantidium coli*.
    iv. *Schistosomal dysentery*: It occurs due to *schistosoma mansonni*, e.g. ipecacuanha.

Q 21. Give synonyms, biological source, chemical constituents and uses of ipecacuanha. (S. 99, 00, 01, 02, 03, 07; W. 01, 02)

Ipecacuanha

- *Synonyms*: Ipecac.
- *Biological source*: It consists of dried roots of the rhizomes and roots of cephalis ipecacuanha A. rich or of cephalis acuminata karsten.
- *Family*: Rubiaceae.
- *Chemical constituents*: It contains:
  i. Isoquinoline alkaloids
  ii. Emetine, cephaeline
  iii. Psychotrine
  iv. O-methyl psychotrine
  v. Emetamine
  vi. Ipecacuantic acid
  vii. Starch and calcium oxalate.
- *Uses*:
  i. It is used as expectorant in small doses and emetic in higher doses
  ii. It is used in treatment of diarrhoea and dysentery
  iii. Used for isolation of emetine and cephaeline.

M DIURETICS

Q 22. What are diuretics? Give examples. (S. 98, 99, 01, 02, 03, 05, 06, 07; W. 98, 99, 04, 05, 06)

Diuretics are the drugs which increase the rate of urine flow, e.g. a. Gokharu, b. Punarnava.

Q 23. Give synonyms, biological source, chemical constituents and uses of drugs: a. Gokharu, b. Punarnava.

a. Gokharu (S. 03; W. 97, 01, 02)

- *Synonym*: Puncture vine.
- *Biological source*: It consists of dried fully ripen fruits of the plant Tribulus terrestries linn.
- *Family*: Zygophyllaceae.
- *Chemical constituents:* It contains:
  i. Harmine and harman

   ii. Steroidal sapogenins like diosgenin
   iii. Gitogenin
   iv. Chlorogenin
   v. Rusogenin
   vi. Kaemferol
   vii. Tribuloside.
- *Uses*:
   i. Used as diuretic, tonic.
   ii. In treatment of calculous affections.
   iii. In treatment of painful micturition.
   iv. Used as aphrodiasic and in gout.

b. Punarnava (S. 03)

- *Synonyms*: Hog weed, Rakto punarnava, Lalsabuni
- *Biological source*: It consists of fresh, as well as dried herbs Boerhaavia diffusa linn.
- *Family*: Nyctaginaceae.
- *Chemical constituents*:
   i. Purarnavine
   ii. Punernavoside
   iii. Potassium nitrate
   iv. Ursolic acid
- *Uses*:
   i. It is used as diuretic and expectorant
   ii. It is stomochic and is used in treatment of jaundice.

N ANTISEPTICS AND DISINFECTANTS

Q 24. What are antiseptics and disinfectants? Give examples. (S. 96, 97, 98, 00, 02, 06, 07, 08; W. 03, 04)

Antiseptics: These are the chemical sterilizing substances which are used to kill pathogenic microbes or for prevention of their growth, e.g. Benzoin, Myrrh, Neem, Curcuma.

Q 25. Give synonyms, biological source, chemical constituents and uses of drugs. a. Benzoin, b. Myrrh, c. Neem, d. Curcuma.

a. Benzoin (S. 97, 99, 06; W. 97, 00, 03)

- *Synonyms*: Sumatra benzoin, Gum benzoin, Loban.
- *Biological source*: Benzoin is a balsamic resin obtained from styrax benzoin dry and or styrax poralleloneurus perkins and other

specifics of styrax known in market as sumatra benzoin or it contains balsamic resin from styrox tonkinesis known as siam benzoin.

- *Family*: Styraceae.
- *Chemical constituents*: It contains:
  - i. Balsamic acid and esters
  - ii. Caniferyl alcohol
  - iii. Coniferyl benzoate
  - iv. Benzoic acid
  - v. Cinnamic acid
  - vi. Sumaresinolic acid.
- *Uses*:
  - i. It is used as irritating expectorant, carminative and diuretic.
  - ii. Externally used as an antiseptic and protective.
  - iii. In treatment of upper respiratory tract infection.
  - iv. Used in soaps, perfumes.

b. Myrrh (S. 02)

- *Synonyms*: Gum myrrh, Bol myrrh.
- *Biological source*: Myrrh is an oleo-gum-resin obtained from cammiphora molmol Engler and from other commiphora species.
- *Family*: Burseraceae.
- *Chemical constituents*: It contains:
  - i. Resin 25 to 40%
  - ii. α, β and γ camphoric acids
  - iii. Terpenes
  - iv. Eugenol
  - v. Cuminic aldehyde
  - vi. Volatile oil.
- *Uses*:
  - i. It is used as an antiseptic and stimulant.
  - ii. It is astringent to the mucous membrane
  - iii. Its tincture is used in the mouthwashes and gargles.

c. Neem (S. 96, 99, 00, 03, 06, 07; W. 99, 05)

- *Synonyms*: Limb, Morgosa, Melia azadirachta.
- *Biological source*: It consists of leaves and other aerial parts of Azadirachta indica.

- *Family*: Meliaceae.
- *Chemical constituents*:
    i. Azadirachtin
    ii. Salannin
    iii. Meliantriol
    iv. Nimbosterol, Nimbiol
    v. Quercetin
    vi. Nimbidinine, Nimaton
    vii. Myrecetin
    viii. Diterpenes (sugiol, nimbiol)
- *Uses*:
    i. It is used as insect repellant, insecticide.
    ii. It has antifeedant and antimicrobial properties.
    iii. Seed oil has spermicidal activity.

d. Turmeric (Curcuma) (S. 98, 99, 00, 02, 03, 06, 07; W. 98, 99)

- *Synonyms*: Haldi, Indian saffron.
- *Biological source*: Turmeric consists of dried as well as fresh rhizomes of the plant known as curcuma longes linn.
- *Family*: Zingiberaceae.
- *Chemical constituents*: It contains:
    i. Curcumin
    ii. Curcuminoids
    iii. Zingiberene
    iv. α and β curcumenes
    v. Comphor
    vi. Camphene
    vii. Volatile oil.
- *Uses*:
    i. It is used as condiment, colouring agent
    ii. It is used for the detection of boric acid
    iii. It is used especially for ointment and creams.

O ANTIMALARIALS

Q 26. What are antimalarials? Give examples. (S. 06)

Antimalarials: These are the drugs which are used in prophylaxis or treatment of malaria, e.g. cinchona.

Malaria occurs due to infections by four species of a protozoan—
Plasmodium species, *P. malariae*, *P. vivax*, *P. ovale*, *P. officinales*.

Q 27. Give synonyms, biological source, chemical constituents and uses of cinchona.

Cinchona (S. 98, 99, 00, 01, 03, 06; W. 98, 99, 00)

- *Synonyms*: Jesuit's bark, Peruvian bark.
- *Biological source*: It is the dried bark of cultivated trees of cinchona calisaya wedd, c. ledgeriana moens, cinchona officinalis linn.
- *Family*: Rubiaceae.
- *Chemical constituents*: It contains:
    - i. Quinine
    - ii. Quinidine
    - iii. Cinchonine
    - iv. Cinchonidine
    - v. Cinchonicine hydroquinine
    - vi. Quinicine.
- *Uses*:
    - i. It is used as antimalarial in nature
    - ii. It is employed as bitter stomachic and antipyretics
    - iii. Quinidine is used in prevention of atrial fibrillation
    - iv. Used to arrhythmia and tachycardia.

P OXYTOCICS

Q 28. What are oxytocics? Give examples. (S. 96, 05, 06, 07, 08; W. 98, 01, 02, 03, 04)

Oxytocics: These are the drugs which have stimulant effect on the motility of the uterus, e.g. ergot alkaloid.

Q 29. Give synonyms, biological source, chemical constituents and uses of ergot.

Ergot (S. 96, 97, 98, 99, 00, 01, 03, 06, 08; W. 00, 99)

- *Synonyms*: Ergota, Ergot of Rye.
- *Biological source*: Ergot is the dried sclerotium of a fungus claviceps purpurea.
- *Family*: Hypocreaceae.

- *Chemical constituents*
    i. Ergotamine
    ii. Ergocristine, Ergocryptine
    iii. Ergometrine
    iv. Ergotaminine
    v. Ergosinine
    vi. Ergocorninine.
- *Uses*:
    i. As oxytocic.
    ii. Ergotamine is used in treatment of migraine.
    iii. It is used in labour to assist delivery to reduce postpartum haemorrhage.

Q VITAMINS

Q. 30. What are vitamins? Give examples. (S. 06)

Vitamins: These are the substances which are required for normal growth and maintenance of life of animals, e.g. shark liver oil, amla.

Q 31. Give synonyms, biological source, chemical constituents and uses of shark liver oil.

a. Shark Liver Oil (S. 96, 98, 99, 01, 03; W. 96, 02)

- *Synonyms*: Oleum selachoids.
- *Biological source*: Shark liver oil is the fixed oil obtained from the fresh and carefully preserved livers of various species of the shark.
- *Order:* Selachi
- *Chemical constituents*: It contains vitamin A and fatty acid.
- *Uses*:
    i. It is used as a source of vitamin A and fatty acid
    ii. It is nutritive
    iii. It is used in burn and sunburn
    iv. It is also known as antixerophthalmic factor.

b. Amla (S. 04, 05, 06, 07)

- *Synonyms*: Emblica, Embelic myrobalan.
- *Biological source*: It consists of dried as well as fresh fruits of the plant *Emblica officinalis*.

- *Family*: Euphorbiaceae.
- *Chemical constituents*:
    i. Vitamin C
    0.5% fat
    Phyllemblin
    5% tannin
    Pectin.
    Other inorganic constituents are iron, calcium, phosphorus.
- *Uses*:
    i. In the treatment of scruvy.
    ii. It is used as a diuretic laxative.
    iii. Fruits are given in diarrhoea and dysentery.
    iv. They are administered in jaundice, anaemia alongwith iron compound.
    v. It is given in treatment of asthma and bronchitis.

R ENZYMES

Q 32. What are enzymes? Give examples. (S. 96, 99; W. 99)

Enzymes are the protein substances, which serve a role of catalysing the biochemical reactions in living systems, e.g. diastase, yeast, papaya.

Q 33. Give synonyms, biological source, chemical constituents and uses of: a. Diastase, b. Yeast, c. Papaya.

a. Diastase (S. 96)

- *Synonyms*: Amylose, malt diastase, salivary diastase.
- *Biological source*: It is one of the amylotyic enzymes present in saliva found in digestive tract of the animals (animal diastase).
- *Family*: Gramineae
- *Description*:
    i. It is yellowish white
    ii. It has faint characteristic odour
    iii. It is soluble in water forms collodial solution.
- *Uses*:
    i. It is used as digestant.
    ii. Used as catalyse reactions in plant and animal.

b. Yeast

Yeast is a fungi which under normal conditions of growth, contains a vegetative body of simple individual cell.

- *Biological source*: It consists of unicellular fungal microorganisms, *Saccharomyces cerevisiae*.
- *Family*: Saccharomycetaceae.
- *Description*:
  - i. *Colour*: Whitish powder
  - ii. *Odour*: Characteristic
  - iii. *Size*: Unicellular microorganism range less than 1.5 μ.
- *Chemical constituents*: It contains:
  - i. Glycogen, fat and vitamins
  - ii. Thiamine, riboflavin, nicotinic acid
  - iii. Folic acid, biotin
  - iv. Enzymes like invertase, diastase, zymase.
- *Uses*:
  - i. Used in manufacture of alcohol, beer and wines.
  - ii. In bread industry.
  - iii. Used as source of vitamin D.
  - iv. It is a good source of pr' tein.

c. Papaya (S. 99, 00, 02, 06, 07; W. 02)

- *Biological source*: It is cultivated fruiting tree known as carica papaya linn.
- *Family*: Caricaceae.
- *Description*:
  Colour—light brown or white coloured amorphous powder
  Odour and taste is typical
  pH—5 to 6.1
- *Solubility*: Soluble in water and glycerine.
- *Chemical constituents*:
  - i. Chymopapain
  - ii. Polypeptides
  - iii. Amides.
- *Uses*:
  - i. Used in clarification of beverages
  - ii. It is used as digestant and anti-inflammatory agent
  - iii. It is used in textile and leather industry for dehairing of skins and hides.

S PERFUMES AND FLAVOURING AGENTS

Q 34. What are perfumes ? Give examples. (S. 96, 98, 07, 08; W. 02)

Perfumes: It is any substance which is made from natural or synthetic materials or a combination of both, employed for creating a pleasant odour, e.g. sandal wood oil.

Flavouring agents: These are the substances which are used to give a flavour to the pharmaceutical formulations, e.g. lemon oil, mint, orange, clove, lavendor, rose, peppermint oil.

Q. 35. Give synonyms, biological source, chemical constituents and uses of following drugs: a. Peppermint oil, b. Sandal wood, c. Lemon oil, d. Orange oil, e. Lemon grass oil.

a. Peppermint Oil (S. 07; W. 04)

- *Synonyms*: Oleum, Mentha piperita.
- *Biological source*: Peppermint oil is the volatile oil obtained by steam distillation of the fresh flowering tops of the plant known as Mentha piperita linn.
- *Family*: Labiatae.
- *Chemical constituents*:
  - i. L-menthol
  - ii. Menthone
  - iii. Methyl acetate
  - iv. Terpene derivatives include L-limonene, cineole, pinene, camphene, isopulegone.
- *Uses*:
  - i. It is used as carminative, aromatic.
  - ii. Stimulant.
  - iii. Counter irritant.
  - iv. Flavouring agent.
  - v. It has antiseptic property.
  - vi. Used in jellies, candles, perfumes.
  - vii. Used in toothpaste and powder, shaving creams.

b. Sandal Wood (S. 05; W. 03, 05)

- *Synonyms*: Yellow sandal wood, lignum santali.
- *Biological source*: It is the dried heartwood of santalum album linn.

- *Family*: Santalaceae.
- *Chemical constituents*:
    i. α-santalol
    ii. β-santalol
    iii. Santalal
    iv. Santene
    v. Santenone
    vi. Teresantol.
- *Uses*:
    i. As a perfume in cosmetics and incense sticks.
    ii. For the treatment of dysuria.
    iii. For carvings and manufacture of boxes.

c. **Lemon Oil (S. 98, 07; W. 00)**

- *Biological source*: Lemon oil is a volatile oil obtained from the fresh peel of the ripe fruits of citrus-lemon.
- *Family*: Rutaceae.
- *Chemical constituents*:
    i. Lemonene
    ii. Citral
    iii. Citronellal.
- *Uses*:
    i. Flavouring agent
    ii. In perfumery.

d. **Orange Oil (S. 96)**

- *Synonyms*: Sweet orange oil, oleum auranti.
- *Biological source*: Orange is the volatile oil obtained from orange peels of sweet orange of citrus-sinensis.
- *Family*: Rutaceae.
- *Chemical constituents*:
    i. Limonene
    ii. Cetronellal
    iii. Citral
    iv. Decanal.

e. **Lemon Grass Oil (S. 96; W. 02, 03)**

- *Synonyms*: East Indian lemon grass oil.
- *Biological source*: It is a volatile oil obtained from the leaves and aerial parts of the plants cymbopogon flexuosus.

- *Family*: Graminae.
- *Chemical constituents*:
    i. Citral
    ii. Methylheptenol
    iii. Nerol
    iv. Geraniol.
- *Uses*:
  i. Flavouring agent
  ii. In perfumery.

T PHARMACEUTICAL AIDS

Q 36. Define and classify pharmaceutical aids with examples. (S. 97, 98, 99, 02, 03, 04, 05, 06, 07, 08; W. 98, 99, 01, 06, 07)

- *Pharmaceutical aids*: The substances which are of little or no therapeutic value, but are essentially used in manufacturing or compounding of various pharmaceuticals are known as pharmaceutical aids.
- *Classification*: (As per use of application)
    i. *Colour*: Caramel, saffron, indigo
    ii. *Diluent*: Cinnamon water, sesame oil
    iii. *Disintegrating agent*: Starch, CMC
    iv. *Emulsifying*: Acacia, tragacanth and suspending agent
    v. *Flavours*: Cardamom, rose, cinnamon
    vi. *Lubricants*: Talc, cocoa butter
    vii. *Ointment bases*: Beeswax, lanolin
    viii. *Solvents*: Alcohol, glycerine
    ix. *Sweetening agents*: Honey, sorbitol.

Q 37. Give synonyms, biological source, chemical constituents and uses of following drugs: a. Acacia, b. Guar gum, c. Honey, d. Starch, e. Tragacanth f. Agar, g. Arachis oil, h. Olive oil, i. Lanolin.

a. Acacia Indian Gum (S. 06)

- *Synonyms*: Gum acacia, Gum arabic.
- *Biological source*: Indian gum is the dried gummy exudation obtained from the stem and branches of acacia arabica wild.
- *Family*: Leguminosae.

- *Chemical constituents*:
    i. Arabin
    ii. Arabic acid
    iii. Enzyme-oxidase.
- *Uses*:
    i. Demulcent
    ii. Suspending agent
    iii. Emulsifying agent
    iv. Binding agent
    v. As a gum of choice.

b. **Guar gum**

- *Synonyms*: Guar flour, Jaguar gum.
- *Biological source*: Guar gum is the powder of endosparm of seeds of cyamopsis tetragonolobus.
- *Family*: Leguminosae.
- *Chemical constituents*:
    i. Guaran
    ii. 5–7% proteins.
- *Uses*:
    i. Binding and disintegrating agent
    ii. Bulk laxative
    iii. Appetite depressant
    iv. In peptic ulcer therapy
    v. In paper manufacturing, printing
    vi. In food and cosmetic industries.

c. **Honey (S. 98, 00, 01, 03, 04, 06; W. 02, 04)**

- *Synonyms*: Madhu, honey purified, mel.
- *Biological source*: Honey is a sugar secretion deposited in honey comb by the bees Apis mellifica, Apis dorsata.
- *Family*: Hymenoptera.
- *Chemical constituents*:
    i. Glucose, fructose and sucrose
    ii. Maltose
    iii. Gum
    iv. Traces of succinic acid.

- *Uses*:
    - i. Demulscent
    - ii. Sweetening agent
    - iii. Good nutrient
    - iv. Antiseptic
    - v. Ingredient of common cough mixtures, cough drops
    - vi. In preparation of creams, soft drinks, candles.

d. Starch (S. 00, 01; W. 98, 00)

- *Synonyms*: Amylum.
- *Biological source*: Starch consists of polysaccharide granules obtained from the grains of maize, rice or wheat.
- *Family*: Gramineae.
- *Chemical constituents*
    - i. α-amylose
    - ii. β-amylose
    - iii. Amylopectin.
- *Uses*:
    - i. Nutritive
    - ii. Demulcent
    - iii. Protective
    - iv. Absorbent
    - v. Antidote in iodine poisoning
    - vi. Disintegrating agent in tablets and pills
    - vii. In preparations of dusting talcum powder.

e. Tragacanth (S. 96; W. 01)

- *Synonyms*: Tragacantha, gum tragacanth.
- *Biological source*: Tragacanth is the dried gummy exudation obtained by making incisions on stems and branches of Astragalus gummifer.
- *Family:* Leguminosae.
- *Chemical constituents*:
    - i. Tragacanthin
    - ii. Bassorin
    - iii. Tragacanthic acid.
- *Uses*:
    - i. Demulscent and emollient in cosmetics
    - ii. Also used in confectionery

iii. Thickening, suspending and emulsifying agent

iv. Binding agent and excipient in the pills.

f. Agar

- *Synonyms*: Agar-agar, Japanese-isinglass.
- *Biological source*: It is the dried gelatinous substance obtained from Gelidium amansii.
- *Family*: Rhodophyceae.
- *Chemical constituents*:
  i. Agarose
  ii. Agaropectin.
- *Uses*:
  i. Emulsifying agent
  ii. Bulk laxative
  iii. In preparation of jellies, confectionery items
  iv. Used in culture medium.

g. Arachis Oil

- *Synonyms*: Ground nut oil, peanut oil.
- *Biological source*: It is a fixed oil expressed from the seed Kernels of the activated varieties of Arachis hypogea.
- *Family*: Leguminosae.
- *Chemical constituents*:
  i. Oleic acid
  ii. Linoleic acid
  iii. Stearic acid
  iv. Arachidic acid
  v. Lignoceric acid
  vi. Palmitic acid.
- *Uses*
  i. As a solvent for intramuscular injections
  ii. In preparation of liniments and soaps
  iii. As a lubricants
  iv. As a edible oil.

h. Olive Oil

- *Synonyms*: Oleum olivae.
- *Biological source*: It is a fixed oil expressed from the ripe fruit of olea europoea.

- *Family*: Oleaceae.
- *Chemical constituents*:
    i. Olein
    ii. Palmitin
    iii. Linolein.
- *Uses*:
    i. Emollient
    ii. Soothing agent
    iii. In psoriasis
    iv. As a nutritive, demulcent
    v. Mild laxative.

i. Lanolin (Hydrous Wool Fat) (S. 02, 03, 09; W. 04, 08)

- *Synonyms*: Lanolin, Adeps lanae.
- *Biological source*: Hydrous wool fat is the purified fat-like substance obtained from the wool of the sheeps oris aries.
- *Family*: Boridae.
- *Chemical constituents*:
    i. Esters of cholesterol and isocholesterol
    ii. 50% of water.
- *Uses*:
    i. As a water absorbable ointment base
    ii. As a base for water soluble creams and cosmetic preparations.

j. Beeswax (S. 96; W. 01, 02)

- *Synonyms*: Yellow beeswax.
- *Biological source*: Yellow beeswax is purified wax and obtained from honey comb of the bees Apis mellifeca.
- *Family*: Apidae
- *Chemical constituents*:
    i. Myricin (myricyl palmitate)
    ii. Cerotic acid
    iii. Cerolein
- *Uses*:
    i. Used in preparation of ointments, plasters and polishes.
    ii. Used in manufacture of candles, moulds, lipsticks, face creams, etc.

U MISCELLANEOUS DRUGS

Q. 38. Give synonyms, biological source, chemical constituents and uses of following drugs: a. Liquorice, b. Picrorriza, c. Linseed oil, d. Shatavari, e. Shankhpushpi, f. Garlic, g. Tobacco, h. Dioscorea, i. Pyrethrum.

a. **Liquorice (S. 99, 01, 03; W. 97, 00)**

- *Synonyms*: Liquorice root, Glycyrrhiza, Mulethi, Jasthi-Madhu.
- *Biological source*: Liquorice consists of dried peeled or unpeeled roots and stolons of the plant known as glycyrrhiza glabra linn.
- Family: Leguminosae.
- *Chemical constituents*: It contains:
    i. Glycyrrhizin
    ii. Glycyrrhizinic acid
    iii. Glycyrrhetinic acid
    iv. Flavone glycoside
    v. Liquiritin glucose
    vi. Asparagine (2 to 4%) and fat.
- *Uses*:
    i. It is used as demulcent and mild expectorant
    ii. It is used as flavouring agent, antispasmodic
    iii. In treatment of Addison's disease
    iv. In treatment of peptic ulcer and anti-inflammatory agent.

b. **Picrorriza (S. 04)**

- *Synonyms*: Katki, Kadu, Indian gentian, Kutki.
- *Biological source*: It consists of dried rhizomes of the plant picrorrhiza kurroa.
- *Family*: Scrophulariaceae.
- *Chemical constituents*:
    i. Picroside I
    ii. Picroside II
    iii. Kutkoside
    iv. Vanilloyl
    v. Trans-cinnamoyl.
- *Uses*:
    i. It is used as bitter tonic, stomachic
    ii. It is laxative

    iii. In treatment of jaundice

    iv. It has antibacterial effect.

c. Linseed Oil (S. 98, 99, 01; W. 00)

- *Synonyms*: Flax seed, Linum, Jovas.
- *Biological source*: It consists of fixed oil obtained from the dried fully ripe seeds of the linum usitatassimum linn.
- *Family*: Linaceae.
- *Chemical constituents*:
   - i. Palmitic acid
   - ii. Stearic acid
   - iii. Oleaic acid
   - iv. Linoleic and linolenic acid
   - v. Tocopherol and squalene.
- *Uses*:
   - i. It is mainly for external applications as lotion and liniments
   - ii. It is used in treatment of scabies and skin diseases
   - iii. It is nutritive and emollient
   - iv. Used for paints and varnishes.

d. Shatavari (S. 03)

- *Synonyms*: Shatmuli.
- *Biological source*: It consists of dried roots and leaves of the plant known as Asparagus racemosus wild.
- *Family*: Liliaceae.
- *Chemical constituents*:
   - i. Shatavarin-I, II, III, IV
   - ii. Sarsapogenin
   - iii. Rhamnose moieties.
- *Uses*:
   - i. Used as galactogogue, tonic, diuretic
   - ii. In treatment of rheumatism and nervin disorder
   - iii. It is used in Ayurveda in threatened, abortion.

e. Shankhpushpi (S. 96)

- *Synonyms*: Shankhvel, Shankhphuli.
- *Biological source*: It consists of the aerial parts of the plant known as canscora decussata.
- *Family*: Gentianaceae.

- *Chemical constituents*:
    i. It contains oleo-resin
    ii. Triterpenes
    iii. Alkaloids
    iv. Xanthones.
- *Uses*:
    i. It is used as bitter, nervine tonic
    ii. In treatment of epilepsy, nervous debility.

f. Garlic (S. 99; W. 99)

- *Synonyms*: Allium, Lasun, Lasan.
- *Biological source*: It consists of bulbs of the plant known as Allium sativum linn.
- *Family*: Liliaceae.
- *Chemical constituents*:
    i. Carbohydrates 29%
    ii. Allilin
    iii. Allicin
    iv. Allyl propyl disulphide
    v. Diallyl disulphide.
- *Uses*:
    i. It is used as carminative, expectorant, aphrodiasic.
    ii. Used as anthelmintic, rubefacient.
    iii. It is useful in high blood pressure and atherosclerosis.
    iv. It is used as condiment.
    v. It has antibacterial.
    vi. It posses cholesterol suppressing property.

g. Tobacco (S. 98, 02; W. 97)

- *Synonyms*: Tambaku, Tamak, tumbakhu.
- *Biological source*: It consists of dried leaves of nicotine tobacco.
- *Family*: Solanoceae.
- *Chemical constituents*:
    i. Nicotine
    ii. Anabasine
    iii. Nornicotine.
- *Uses*:
    i. It is powerful quick acting poison
    ii. It exerts stimulant effect on heart and nervous system.

h. Dioscorea (S. 03; W. 96, 01, 05)

- *Synonym*: Yam.
- *Biological source*: It consists of dried tubers of the plant dioscorea deltoidea and other species of dioscorea.
- *Family*: Dioscoreaceae.
- *Chemical constituents*
  - i. Diosgenin
  - ii. Sapogenin
  - iii. Glycoside
  - iv. Phenolic compounds.
- *Uses*:
  - i. It is used as for several corticosteroids sex hormones
  - ii. Used in oral contraceptives
  - iii. In treatment of rheumatic arthritis.

i. Pyrethrum (S. 98, 99, 02, 03, 08; W. 00)

- *Synonyms*: Natural pyrethum, insect flowers.
- *Biological source*: It consists of dried flower-heads of chrysanthemum cinerariefolium and other species of chrysanthemum.
- *Family*: Compositeae.
- *Chemical constituents*:
  - i. Pyrethrin-I–II
  - ii. Cinerin-I–II
  - iii. Jasmolin-I–II
  - iv. Chrysanthenic acid
  - v. Pyrethric acid
  - vi. Cinerolone
  - vii. Jasmolone.
- *Uses*:
  - i. It is used as insecticide
  - ii. Used in preparation of mosquito coils and insect repellent formulations.

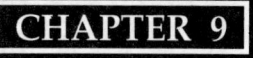

CHAPTER 9

Gross Anatomical Studies of Some Crude Drugs

Q 1. Draw a well labelled diagrammatic TS of following crude drugs.

1. **TS of Senna Leaflet (S. 06, 07)**

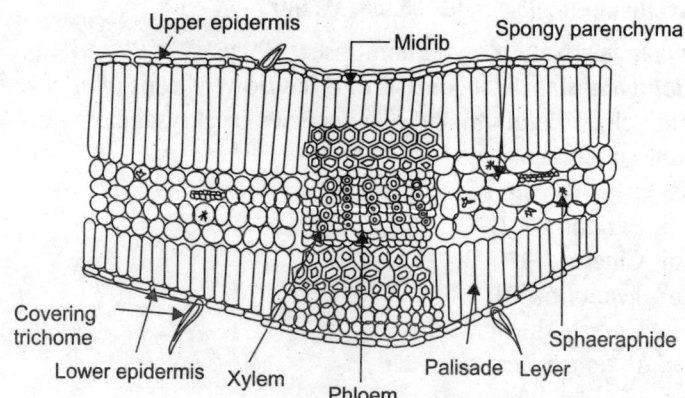

2. **TS of Datura**

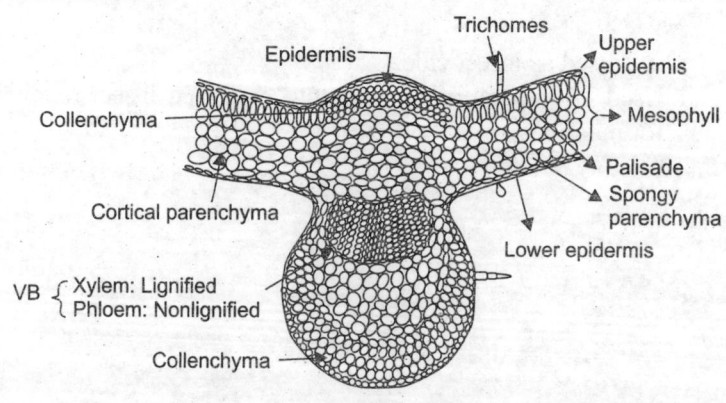

3. TS of Cinnamon Bark (S. 06)

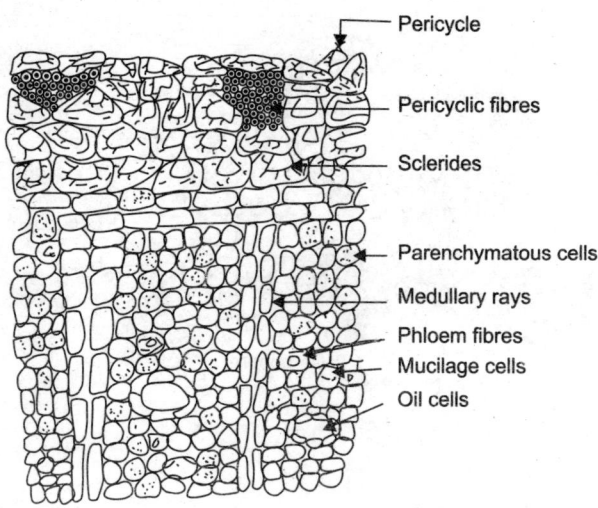

- Pericycle
- Pericyclic fibres
- Sclerides
- Parenchymatous cells
- Medullary rays
- Phloem fibres
- Mucilage cells
- Oil cells

4. TS of Cinchona Bark (S. 04, 07; W. 08)

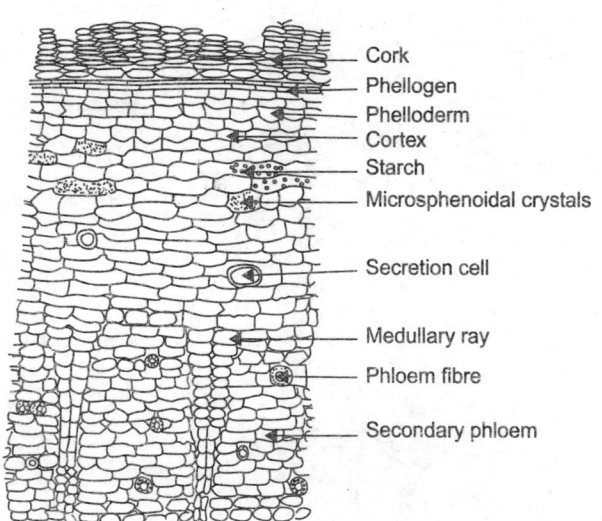

- Cork
- Phellogen
- Phelloderm
- Cortex
- Starch
- Microsphenoidal crystals
- Secretion cell
- Medullary ray
- Phloem fibre
- Secondary phloem

5. TS of Fennel (S. 08)

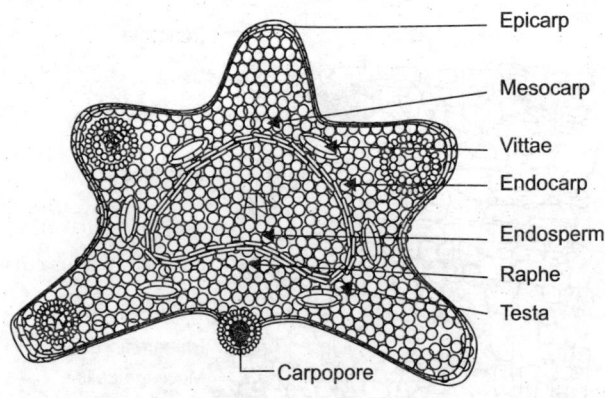

Epicarp

Mesocarp

Vittae

Endocarp

Endosperm

Raphe

Testa

Carpopore

6. TS of Clove

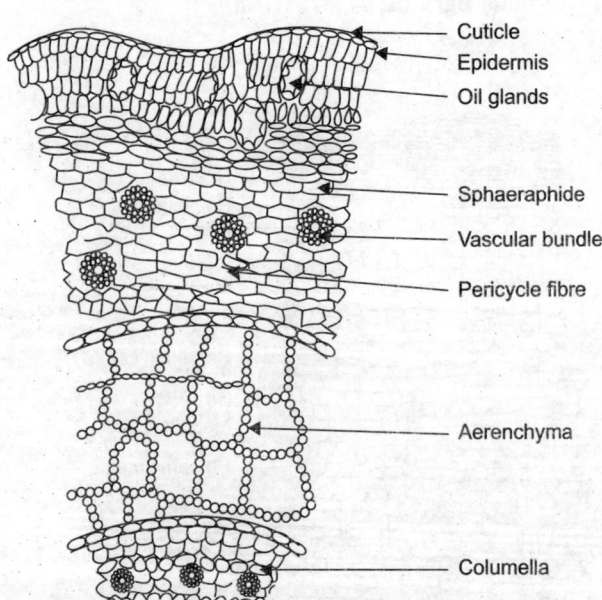

Cuticle

Epidermis

Oil glands

Sphaeraphide

Vascular bundle

Pericycle fibre

Aerenchyma

Columella

7. TS of Ginger (W. 04)

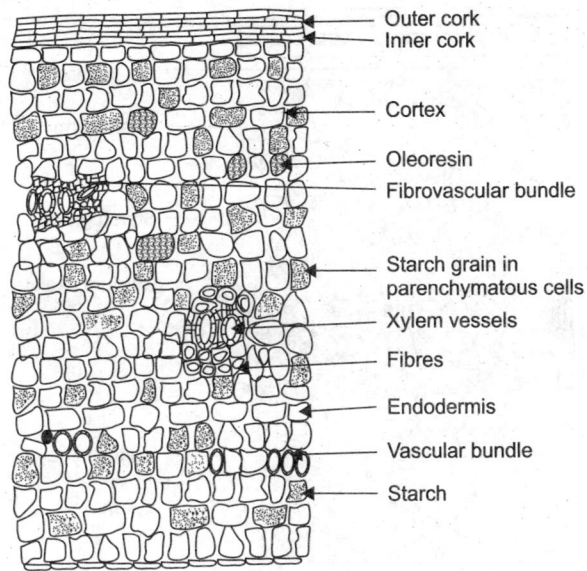

- Outer cork
- Inner cork
- Cortex
- Oleoresin
- Fibrovascular bundle
- Starch grain in parenchymatous cells
- Xylem vessels
- Fibres
- Endodermis
- Vascular bundle
- Starch

8. TS of Nux-vomica Seed (S. 05; W. 07)

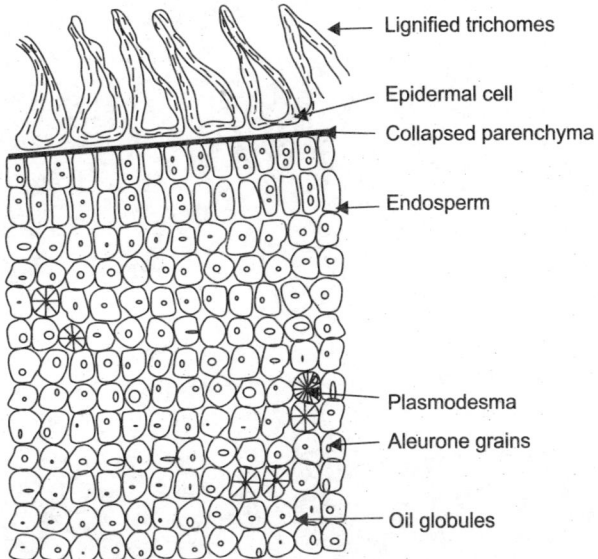

- Lignified trichomes
- Epidermal cell
- Collapsed parenchyma
- Endosperm
- Plasmodesma
- Aleurone grains
- Oil globules

9. TS of Ipecacuanha

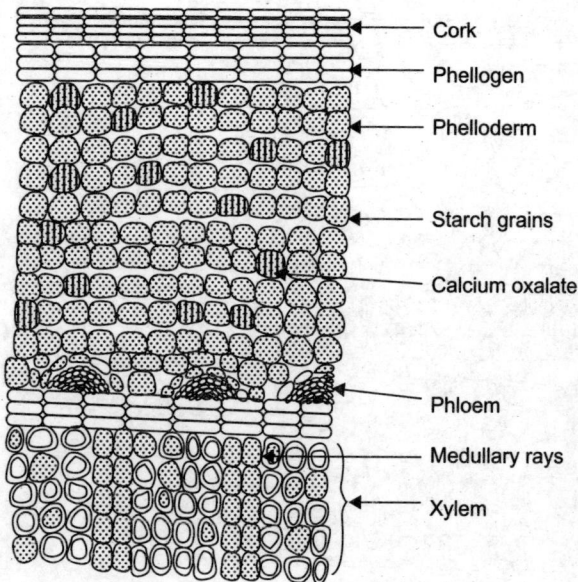

Cork

Phellogen

Phelloderm

Starch grains

Calcium oxalate

Phloem

Medullary rays

Xylem

Appendix

A. Synonymes of Some Crude Drugs

1. Turmeric: Indian saffron
2. Diastase: Amylase
3. Picrorrhiza: Indian gentian
4. Starch: Amylum
5. Vasaka: Adhatoda
6. Nutmeg: Banda soap
7. Tulsi: Sacred basil
8. Digitalis: Foxglove leaves
9. Cinchona: Jesuits bark
10. Senna: Tinnevelly senna
11. Pyrethrum: Insect flowers
12. Nux-vomica: Crow-fig.
13. Aloes: Musabbar, korphad
14. Rhubarb: Radix
15. Vinca: Periwinkle
16. Asafoetida: Devils dung
17. Clove: Caryophyllum
18. Rauwolfia: Sarpagandha
19. Aconite: Bachnag, visha
20. Ephedra: Ma-Hung
21. Gokharu: Puncture vine
22. Dioscorea: Yam
23. Olive oil: Oleum olivae
24. Colchicum: Meadow saffron

25. Agar: Japanese Isinglass
26. Ginger: Zingeber, Ale
27. Ajowan: Carum copiticum hieren
28. Honey: Mel
29. Ashwagandha: Withania root
30. Lanolin: Hydrous wool fat
31. Cinnamon: Kalmi-dalchini
32. Ginger: Zingiber
33. Fennel: Fructus foeniculum
34. Cannabis: Bhang, Indian Hemp.
35. Amla: Indian goose berry
36. Guggul: Indian bdellium
37. Pterocarpus: Malbar kino, Indian kino
38. Liquorice: Mulethi
39. Garlic: Allium, Lasun
40. Shatavari: Shatmuli
41. Shankhapushpi: Shankhvel
42. Linseed: Flax seed
43. Kaolin: China clay
44. Shark liver oil: Oleum selachoids
45. Neem: Margosa
46. Punarnava: Hog weed
47. Gymnema: Gudmar, Madhunashini
48. Hyoscyamus: Henbane
49. Black catechu: Kattha
50. Ispaghula: Indian Psyllium

B. **Parts of the Plant Used as a Drug**

1. Guggul: Oleogum resin
2. Arjuna: Bark
3. Ephedra: Dried young stems
4. Punarnava: Dried herb
5. Digitalis: Leaf
6. Nutmeg: Seed
7. Gymnema: Leaf
8. Pyrethrum: Flower heads
9. Vinca: Leaf
10. Belladonna: Roots
11. Cannabis: Dried flowing and fruiting tops

12. Rhubarb: Rhizome
13. Cardamom: Fruit
14. Rauwolfia: Roots
15. Nux-vomica: Seeds
16. Ginger: Rhizomes
17. Gokharu: Fruit
18. Clove: Flower bud
19. Aconite: Dried root
20. Gelatin: Animal collagen
21. Vasaka: Leaves
22. Shatavari: Dried roots and leaves
23. Aloe: Juice of leaves
24. Senna: Leaflet
25. Black pepper: Fruit
26. Linseed: Seed
27. Liquorice: Roots
28. Coriander: Fruit
29. Fennel: Fruit
30. Garlic: Bulbs
31. Ajowan: Fruit
32. Turmeric: Rhizomes
33. Cinchona bark
34. Ipecacunha: Dried roots and rhizomes
35. Ashwagandha: Roots
36. Isapghulla: Seeds
37. Cardamom: Fruit
38. Hyocyamus: Dried leaves and flowing tops
39. Belladonna: Leaf
40. Tulsi: Fresh and dried leaves

C. **Name the Crude Drugs Containing one of the Following Constituent**

1. Curcumin: Turmeric
2. Quinine: Cinchona
3. Vitamin C: Amla
4. Emetine: Ipecac
5. Fenchone: Fennel
6. Invert sugar: Honey
7. Atropine: Belladonna
8. Reserpine: Rauwolfia

9. Vincristine: Vinca
10. Pyrethrin: Pyrethrum
11. Gingerone: Ginger
12. Chaulmoogric acid: Chaulmoogra oil
13. Cinnamic aldehyde: Cinnamon
14. Shataverin: Shatavari
15. Glycyrrhizin: Liquorice
16. Barbaloin: Aloe
17. Azadirectin: Neem
18. Gumnemic acid: Gymnema
19. Guggulsterone: Guggul
20. Serpentine: Rauwolfia
21. Aconitine: Aconite
22. Withaferin: Ashwagandha
23. Vitamin A: Shark liver A
24. Eugenol: Clove
25. Brucine: Nux-vomica
26. Hydnocarpic acid: Chaulmoogra oil
27. Vasicine: Vasaka
28. Colchicine: Colchicum
29. d-Linalool: Coriander
30. Kutkoside: Picrorrhiza
31. Morphine: Opium
32. Cholesterol: Lanolin
33. Rhein: Senna
34. Arabin: Acacia
35. Myricin: Nutmeg
36. Linamarin: Linseed
37. Scopolamine: Datura
38. Piperine: Black pepper
39. Allicine: Garlic
40. Aldobionic acid: Isapghulla
41. Kino red: Pterocarpus
42. Sennoside A and B: Senna
43. Agarose: Agar
44. Kutkin: Picrorrhiza
45. Bassorin: Tragacanth
46. Oleo-gum-resin: Guggul
47. Digoxin: Digitalis

48. Arjunine: Arjuna
49. Emodin: Rhubarb
50. Diosogenin: Dioscorea
51. Catechin: Pale catechu
52. Ricinolic acid: Castor oil
53. Limonene: Lemon oil
54. Zingiberene: Ginger
55. Cannabidol: Cannabis
56. Ergometrine: Ergot
57. Ephedrine: Ephedra
58. Vasicinone: Vasaka
59. Capsaicin: Capsicum
60. Sinigrin: Mustard

Board Question Papers

(From Summer 1996 to Summer 2017)

Summer Examination 1996
D Pharm First Year
Pharmacognosy

Q 1. Answer any *five* of the following:

    a. Define the following terms giving one example of a crude drug each.
   - i. Antitumour
   - ii. Disinfectants

    b. Describe how Galen contributed in development of pharmacognosy.

    c. Match the following:

i. Turmeric	1. Amylum
ii. Diastase	2. Amylase
iii. Picrorrhiza	3. Indian saffron
iv. Starch	4. Indian gentian

    d. Name any two crude drugs showing laxative property along with responsible active consituent.

    e. Draw a well-labelled diagram of the TS of fennel.

    f. Differentiate between fixed oil and volatile oil.

Q 2. Answer any *four* of the following:

    a. Describe why extractive values are useful in evaluation of crude drugs.

    b. Define flavouring agents. Name any two drugs, which are used as flavouring agents.

    c. Describe in brief, how digitalis is collected and prepared for the market to meet the pharmacopoeial standards.

    d. Describe the chemical method of classification of crude drugs along with its advantages and disadvantages.

e. Give the biological source and uses of absorbent cotton.

f. What are tannins? Give the general chemical tests for tannins.

Q 3. Answer any *four* of the following:

a. Define:
   i. Astringents   ii. Official title

b. Write a note on 'Indigenous system of medicine.'

c. What are vitamins? Give chemical constituents of shark liver oil.

d. Give the uses of:
   i. Shankhapuspi   ii. Beeswax

e. Give the diagnostic characters of coriander.

f. Write a short note on antihypertensives.

Q 4. Answer any *four* of the following:

a. Prepare a note on chemical assay methods.

b. Name the family to which following drugs belong:
   i. Lemon grass oil
   ii. Black pepper
   iii. Neem

c. Explain 'drying' in preparation of crude drug for market.

d. How stomata and trichomes help in the evaluation of crude drugs.

e. What are sutures? How are they sterilized?

f. What are resins? How are they classified?

Q 5. Answer any *four* of the following:

a. What are umbelliferous fruits? Give two examples.

b. Define the terms:
   i. Technical use
   ii. Oxytocics

c. Name any two drugs having antirheumatic property.

d. Give the biological source of following drugs:
   i. Tragacanth
   ii. Agar

e. What are enzymes? Give the uses of diastase.

f. Give the chemical constituents of following drugs.
   i. Ginger
   ii. Orange oil

Q 6. Give the chemical tests for identification of any *four* of the following:

a. Asafoetida   d. Nux vomica

b. Senna   e. Cinnamon

c. Pectin   f. Shark liver oil

Winter Examination 1996
D Pharm First Year
Pharmacognosy

Q 1. Answer any *five* of the following:

a. Define the term pharmacognosy.

b. Write the various sources of crude drugs.

c. Give methods of classification of crude drugs.

d. Who wrote the "Analecta pharmacognostica"?

e. Define adulteration.

f. Name two cardiotonic drugs.

g. Name two drugs belonging to Liliaceae family.

h. Define the term astringent with examples.

Q 2.

a. Write the chemical constituents and uses of following drug (any *four*):

i. Pale catechu	iv. Asafoetida
ii. Aconite	v. Nutmeg
iii. Ashwagandha	vi. Castor oil

b. Match the following:

i. Adhatoda	1. Amla
ii. Benzoin	2. Curcuma longa
iii. Curcumin	3. Vasaka
iv. Quinine	4. Cinnamic acid
v. Vitamin C	5. Starch
vi. Amylose	6. Cinchona

Q 3.

a. What are alkaloids? Give general properties and tests for alkaloids.

b. Describe with a neat-labelled diagram of the TS of unpeeled ginger.

Q 4.

a. Name three drugs belonging to family solanaceae and write their chemical constituents.

b. What is mean by evaluation of crude drugs? Explain morphological evaluation.

Q 5. Write the biological sources and uses of following (any *four*):

a. Ephedra	d. Ergot
b. Vinca	e. Digitalis
c. Shark liver oil	f. Dioscorea

Q 6.

    a. What are sutures and ligatures? Classify with examples.

    b. Give the chemical tests for any two of the following:

        i. Senna   iii. Black catechu

        ii. Nux-vomica

Summer Examination 1997
D Pharm First Year
Pharmacognosy

Q 1. Answer any *four* of the following:

    a. Define:

        i. Astringent   ii. Antiseptic

    b. Mention which part of the plant is useful as a drug in case of:

        i. Cinnamon   iii. Nux-vomica

        ii. Fennel   iv. Rhubarb

    c. Why cascara bark should be stored one year before use?

    d. Define pharmaceutical aids.

    e. Name the different methods of drug evaluation.

    f. Give two examples of crude drugs each from Apocyanaceae, Liliaceae.

    g. Define carminative with examples.

Q 2.

    a. Give the histology, chemical constituents and uses of nux-vomica.

    b. Define pharmacognosy. Who wrote the book "Pharmacognostica gignostica"?

                                Or

    Name the important chemical constituents and give chemical tests for benzoin.

Q 3.

    a. Define the term organized and unorganized drug with example. How do you identify them?

    b. Match the following:

i.	Belladonna	1.	Vasaka
ii.	Emetine	2.	Atropine
iii.	Adhatoda	3.	Ipecac
iv.	Rauwolfia	4.	Reserpine
v.	Fenchone	5.	Fennel
vi.	Honey	6.	Invert sugar

Q 4. Following are the active constituents. Give biological source and uses of the drug containing receptive active constituent (any *seven*):

a. Vincristine
b. Pyrethrin
c. Gingerone
d. Chaulmoogric acid
e. Cinnamic aldehyde
f. Shataverin
g. Glycyrrhizin
h. Quinine
i. Barbaloin

Q 5.

a. Describe the collection and preparation of digitalis for market.
b. What are tannins? Give important tests for tannins. Classify tannins with examples.

Q 6.

a. Give the chemical tests for any two of the following:
  i. Clove   iii. Ergot
  ii. Chaulmoogra oil
b. What are sutures, ligatures and surgical dressings? Classify sutures with examples.

Winter Examination 1997
D Pharm First Year
Pharmacognosy

Q 1. Define pharmacognosy. Name the various sources of drugs. Describe in detail methods of calssification of crude drugs with examples.

Q 2.

a. What do you mean by evaluation of crude drugs? Give methods of drug evaluation. Explain chemical evaluation.
b. Name four drugs containing anthraquinone glycosides. With the biological sources and uses of any two.

Q 3.

a. Describe the histology of nux vomica seed, with neat labelled diagram and give its uses.

b. Answer any two of the following:
  i. What are glycosides? Write identification test for digitalis.
  ii. Give chemical tests for Agar.
  iii. Define technical products with examples.

Q 4. Write biological source, active constituents and uses of the following (any *four*):

a. Fennel   e. Castor oil
b. Rauwolfia   f. Vasaka
c. Gokharu   g. Benzoin
d. Ephedra

Q 5.

a. Define suture, ligatue and surgical dressings. Classify sutures with examples.
b. Write the biological source and active constituents of following:
  i. Tobacco   iii. Liquorice
  ii. Tulsi

Q 6.

a. Match the following:
  i. Shark-liver oil   1. Carminative
  ii. Black pepper   2. Enzyme
  iii. Nux vomica   3. Antitumour
  iv. Yeast   4. Ergot
  v. Vinca   5. Strychnine
  vi. Oxytocic   6. Vitamin A
                             7. Ricinoleic acid
b. Following are active constituents, name the drug, write the biological source and uses (any *four*):
  i. Coriander   iv. Cinnamic aldehyde
  ii. Fibroin   v. Cellulose
  iii. Digoxin   vi. Vincristin

Summer Examination 1998
D Pharm First Year
Pharmacognosy

Q 1.

a. Answer any *five* of the following:
  i. Explain cardiotonics with examples.
  ii. Name the various sources of crude drugs with examples.

    iii. Explain galenical pharmacy and contribution of galen of pharmacy.

    iv. Name the two drugs belonging to family apocyanaceae.

    v. Explain the chemical constituents of one drug, which is used as an anticancer drug.

    vi. Name various methods of classification of crude drugs.

    vii. Define "pharmacognosy" and name the various traditional Indian system of medicine.

    viii. Define antiseptics with examples.

b. Match the following:

1. Reserpine		i.	Cinchona
2. Banda soap		ii.	Benzoin
3. Crow fig		iii.	Tulsi
4. Panama bark		iv.	Enzyme
5. Cinnamic acid		v.	Rauwolfia
6. Sacred basil		vi.	Pterocarpus
7. Papain		vii.	Anthraquinone glycoside
8. Malabar kino		viii.	Nutmeg
9. Senna		ix.	Cardiac glycoside
10. Foxglove leaves		x.	Loganiaceae

Q 2. Answer any *four* of the following:

a. What are alkaloids and give general chemical test for alkaloids?

b. Explain in brief organoleptic evaluation of crude drugs.

c. Explain biological source, chemical constituents and uses of nutmeg.

d. Explain the methods of preparation of absorbent cotton.

e. Give diagnostic features and uses of ashwagandha.

f. Explain vitamins. Give chemical constituents and uses of shark liver oil.

Q 3. Attempt the following (any *two*):

a. Describe with a neat labelled diagram of the TS of cinchona.

b. Write biological sources and uses of the two drugs of the following:

    i. Ephedra   iii. Pyrethrum

    ii. Turmeric

c. What are sutures? Classify it and give requirements as per IP.

Q 4. Write chemical tests for any *three* of the following:

a. Acacia

b. Digitalis

c. Cinchona

d. Turmeric

e. Senna

Q 5. Answer any *four* of the following:

a. Give the biological source of (any *two*):
   i. Cardamon   iii. Tobacco
   ii. Black catechu
b. Name the two drugs having antidysenteric property.
c. Define the following with the example (any *two*):
   i. Antileprotics
   ii. Diuretics
   iii. Flavouring agents
d. Name various fibres obtained from plant sources and give biological source and uses of absorbent cotton.
e. Name various volatile oil containing drugs and give biological source and uses of one drug.
f. Name the two drugs having antitussive properties.

Q 6. Solve any *two* of the following:

a. What do you mean by biological source? Give biological source, uses and chemical constituents of the drug having oxytocic property?
b. Define pharmaceutical aids? Classify with examples and give biological source and uses of honey.
c. Give the name of the family to which following drugs belongs with their uses (any *three*):
   i. Tragacanth   iv. Linseed
   ii. Lemon peel   v. Cinchona
   iii. Colchicum

Winter Examination 1998
D Pharm First Year
Pharmacognosy

Q 1. Solve any *five* of the following:

a. Define alkaloids. Give their classification and general methods of chemical testing.
b. Define any four with examples (one each):
   i. Laxatives   iv. Antitumour
   ii. Vitamins   v. Diuretics
   iii. Oxytocics   vi. Enzymes
c. What is galenical pharmacy? Give contribution of Galen to the pharmacy and name who is called as father of pharmacy.
d. Define pharmaceutical aids and classify them with examples.

e. What are tannins? How are they classified? Give example of each classes.

f. What are surgical dressing and sutures? Explain how surgical cotton is prepared.

g. Give the biological source (any *two*):
   i. Turmeric   iii. Starch
   ii. Nux-vomica

h. Define pharmacognosy. How this word was coined and who wrote the book 'Analecta pharmacognostica'?

Q 2. Solve any *four* of the following:

a. Give biological source, chemical constituents and uses of cinchona.

b. What are astringents? Give examples and explain chemical test for catechu.

c. Name the different methods of drug adulteration.

d. Define drug evaluation. Name various methods of drug evaluation.

e. Give two crude drugs from each of following families (any *two*):
   i. Apocyanaceae   iii. Umbelliferae
   ii. Rutaceae

f. Explain biological source and diagnostic characters of the drug containing vincristin.

Q 3.

a. Describe the collection and preparation of senna for market.

b. Explain classification of crude drugs. What are merits and demerits of chemical system of classification of crude drugs?

Q 4.

a. Name three drugs acting on the central nervous system. Name the various types of opium with its test for identification.

b. Describe organoleptic evaluation of crude drugs considering underground parts of plants.

Or

Explain the terms organised and unorganised crude drugs with two examples of each class.

Q 5.

a. Fill in the blanks:
   i. _____ test is used for identification of anthraquinone glycosides.
   ii. Myristicin is obtained from _____.
   iii. Vasaka belongs to family _____.
   iv. Parquetary arrangement of cells is the diagnostic features of family _____.

    v. Arjuna is used as _____.

    vi. Combination of oil, gum and resin is known as _____.

  b. Explain the gross-anatomical characters of the transverse section of cinchona bark or ipecacuanha root with suitable diagram.

Q 6.

  a. Give biological source and uses of the drugs containing following chemical constituents (any *four*):

    i. Azadiractin   iv. Guggulsterone

    ii. Hydnocarpic acid   v. Serpentine

    iii. Gymnemic acid   vi. Aconitine

  b. Describe the general method of isolation of alkaloids or tannins.

Summer Examination 1999
D Pharm First Year
Pharmacognosy

Q 1.

  a. Match the following:

    i. Guggul   1. Antidiabetics

    ii. Quinine   2. Rauwolfia

    iii. Antitumour   3. Antimalarials

    iv. Reserpine   4. Vinca

    v. Gymnema   5. Antirheumatic

  b. Answer any *five* of the following:

    i. Define alkaloids and how are they classified.

    ii. Explain history of pharmacognosy in brief.

    iii. Give chemical constituents (any *two*):

      1. Benzoin   3. Shark liver oil

      2. Ephedra

    iv. Give synonym of the following:

      1. Senna   3. Pyrethrum

      2. Digitalis

    v. Explain biological source of the two drugs used as a purgative.

    vi. Explain chemical constituents and chemical tests for opium.

    vii. What is meant by evaluation? Explain chemical evaluation of crude drugs.

    viii. Give methods of classification of crude drugs and explain morphological system of classification with their advantages and disadvantages.

Q 2. Answer any *three* of the following:

    a. Give the method of collection and preparation of digitalis for the market.

    b. Define adulteration. Explain in brief various methods of adulteration of crude drugs.

    c. Explain biological sources and uses of any two drugs:
        i. Linseed   iii. Asafoetida
        ii. Ipecacuanha

    d. Name the drug used as a astringent and give its chemical constituents and uses.

    e. Name the drugs acting on CNS and give chemical test and uses of one drug.

Q 3. Solve any *two* of the following:

    a. Describe with a neat and well-labelled diagram of the TS of digitalis/fennel.

    b. What do you mean by sutures and surgical dressings. Give their requirement as per IP and method of preparation of absorbent cotton.

    c. Define oxytocics. Give diagnostic features, chemical constituents, biological source, uses and chemical test for Ergot.

Q 4. Solve any *four* of the following:

    a. Define pharmaceutical aids. Classify it and give examples of each class.

    b. Name the three drugs belonging to family apocyanaceae with their uses.

    c. Chemotaxonomical classification depends on relation between taxonomy and its biogenesis, explain in brief.

    d. Define:
        i. Diuretics   iii. Antitussive
        ii. Vitamins

    e. Write a note on indigenous system of medicine.

    f. Give the uses of following drugs:
        i. Pterocarpus
        ii. Cotton

Q 5. Explain the chemical test for *three* of the following:

    a. Digitalis

    b. Cinchona

    c. Ergot

    d. Senna

    e. Turmeric

Q 6. Answer any *four* of the following:

a. Name the family to which following drugs belongs:
    i. Nux-vomica   iii. Benzoin
    ii. Neem

b. Define volatile oils and how are they classified?

c. Define the following:
    i. Pharmacognosy   ii. Biological source

d. What are enzymes? Give uses of papain.

e. Give the chemical constituent of the following drugs:
    i. Cinnamon   ii. Lahsun

f. Explain diagnostic features and uses of liquorice.

Winter Examination 1999
D Pharm First Year
Pharmacognosy

Q 1. Answer any five of the following:

a. Define pharmacognosy? How this word was coined?

b. Define with examples (any *two*):
    i. Antidiabetics   iii. Enzymes
    ii. Cardiotonics

c. Define antitussives with two examples.

d. Which part of the plant is used as a drug in case of:
    i. Guggul   iii. Ephedra
    ii. Arjuna   iv. Punarnava

e. Explain the term alkaloids with examples.

f. What are methods of isolation of resins?

g. Name the drug, which contains:
    i. Morphine   ii. Gingerol

Q 2.

a. Explain method of preparation of absorbent cotton and how it is identified chemically.

b. How the glycosides are classified? Give examples.

Or

Explain sutures. What are the official requirements of sutures?

Q 3.

a. Give official source, chemical constituents, chemical tests and uses of clove.

b. Define evaluation of crude drugs. Name various types of evaluation and explain chemical evaluation of crude drugs.

Or

Give biological sources, chemical constituents and uses of the following (any *two*):
   i. Tulsi   iii. Neem
   ii. Turmeric

Q 4.

a. Describe the following (any *two*):
   i. Borntrager test for senna.
   ii. Modified borntrager test for aloes.
   iii. Killer-Killiani test for digitoxose.

b. Name two drugs used as (any *four*):
   i. Diuretics   iv. Astringents
   ii. Antitumour   v. Antirheumatics
   iii. Antileprotics   vi. Laxatives

Q 5.

a. Explain resins and resin combinations with suitable examples of each class. Give chemical tests for Asafoetida.

b. Give biological source, chemical constituents, uses and chemical tests of ergot.

Or

How the crude drugs are classified? Give the various methods of classification of crude drugs. Explain morphological classification of crude drugs with merits and demerits.

Q 6.

a. Match the following:
   i. Banda soap   1. Vinca
   ii. Anthraquinone glycoside   2. Astringent
   iii. Vincristine   3. Withania
   iv. Catechu   4. Enzyme
   v. Ashwagandha   5. Senna
   vi. Vitamin C   6. Fennel
   vii. Papaya   7. Nutmeg
   viii. Fenchone   8. Amla

b. Define pharmaceutical aids. How they are classified? Give suitable examples of each type.

Or

Explain diagnostic characters and uses of the following (any *two*):
   i. Garlic   iii. Nux-vomica
   ii. Wool

Summer Examination 2000
D Pharm First Year
Pharmacognosy

Q 1.

a. Attempt any *five* of the following:
   i. Define glycosides and classify it with examples.
   ii. What is Banda soap? Give the biological source of the drug.
   iii. Explain Killer-Killiani test for digitalis.
   iv. Define balsams with examples.
   v. Define diabetes. Name the drug used for its treatment.
   vi. Define disinfectant with suitable examples.
   vii. Explain various types of treatment with its chemical test.

b. Match the following:

   i. Santalum album   1. Shark liver oil
   ii. Curcumin   2. Ashwagandha
   iii. Gymnema   3. Sandal wood
   iv. Withaferin   4. Diabetes
   v. Vitamin A   5. Turmeric

c. Fill up the blanks:
   i. Digitalis belongs to family _____.
   ii. Cinnamic and balsamic acid is present in _____.
   iii. Tulsi is used as _____.
   iv. Crow fig is the synonym of _____.
   v. _____ is used in the treatment of dysentery.

Q 2. Attempt any *two* of the following:

a. Explain the diagnostic features of any drug with their chemical constituents and uses belonging to family umbelliferae.

b. Explain cardiotonics, give chemical constituents, uses, synonym of the drug used as cardiotonics.

c. Describe with a neat and well-labelled diagram of TS of ginger or senna.

Q 3. Attempt any *three* of the following:

a. Explain biological source of cotton and how the surgical cotton is prepared?

b. Define tannins. Give types of tannins and chemical test to differentiate different types of tannins.

c. Explain life cycle of ergot with well-labelled diagram and state their uses.

d. Differentiate between:

    i. Acacia and tragacanth   ii. Oils and fats

Q 4. Attempt any *four* of the following:

a. What do you mean by an alkaloids and how they are classified?

b. Write biological source of the following (any *two*):

    i. Turmeric   iii. Chaulmoogra oil

    ii. Tulsi

c. Give chemical constituents and uses of the following (any *two*):

    i. Ashwagandha   iii. Guggul

    ii. Ipecacuanha

d. Explain modified Borntrager test for aloe with their use.

e. What are sutures? Classify it and give its requirements as per IP.

f. Name the drug used as insecticide, give its biological source, chemical constituent and use.

Q 5. Explain the chemical test for the following (any *four*):

a. Honey   d. Cinchona

b. Agar   e. Asafoetida

c. Starch   f. Black catechu

Q 6. Attempt any *four* of the following:

a. What is adulteration? Give various methods with suitable examples.

b. Explain microscopic methods of drug evaluation.

c. Give methods for identification of fibres.

d. Explain method for collection and preparation for market for senna.

e. Name the various enzymes with their biological source, chemical constituents and its functions.

f. What do you mean by chemotaxonomy? How is it related with phytochemisty?

Winter Examination 2000
D Pharm First Year
Pharmacognosy

Q 1.

a. Attempt any *five* of the following:

    i. How the "pharmacognosy" word coined and who coined it?

    ii. Name the various methods of evaluation of crude drugs.

    iii. Name four drugs used as laxative.

iv. Explain in brief "indigenous system of medicine".

v. Explain astringent, name the drugs used as astringent.

vi. Give biological source of cinchona.

vii. Explain the chemical test for anthraquinone glucoside.

b. Match the pairs:

1. Papain	i. Nux vomica
2. Crow fig	ii. Enzyme
3. Cinnamic acid	iii. Digitalis
4. Cardiotonic	iv. Turmeric
5. Indian saffron	v. Balsams

c. Explain the chemical test and uses of nux-vomica or benzoin.

Q 2. Attempt any *four* of the following:

a. Explain advantages and disadvantages of the morphological method of classification of crude drugs.

b. Explain naturopathy and Yoga.

c. Define pharmacognosy and explain the history of pharmacognosy.

d. Name the drugs belong to family apocyanaceae. State their uses.

e. What are carminatives and gastrointestinal regulators. Name the drugs used for above.

f. What is the significance of pharmacopoeial standards.

Q 3. Attempt any *four* of the following:

a. What do you mean by narcotic drugs. Name some of the drugs used as narcotic and give their uses.

b. Explain resin and resin combination and give chemical test for asafoetida.

c. Explain the organoleptic method for drug evaluation for underground plant parts.

d. Explain the diagnostic features of the drug pyrethrum.

e. What do you mean by antitussive? Give chemical constituents and uses of Tulsi.

f. Explain the drugs used for the treatment of hypertension with their uses.

Q 4. Give the chemical test for following (any *four*):

a. Nux-vomica
b. Acacia
c. Agar
d. Ergot
e. Starch
f. Tragacanth

Q 5. Attempt any *two* of the following:

a. Describe the biological source, synonym, morphology, chemical constituents, uses and TS of the clove.

b. Explain the source, preparation and identification of fibres used in sutures and surgical dressings.

c. Give the biological source, chemical constituents and method of collection and preparation of market of the drug Rauwolfia.

Q 6. Attempt any *four* of the following:

a. Give the diagnostic features of the drug liquorice with their chemical constituents.

b. Give biological source of any two of the following:
   i. Lemon peel   iii. Tragacanth
   ii. Linseed

c. What do you mean by official source, give the biological source and uses of the drug belonging to family Rutaceae.

d. Name the drugs belongs to family as below:
   i. Apidae   iii. Liliaceae
   ii. Hypocreaceae   iv. Rubiaceae

e. What do you mean by enzymes? Explain yeast or diastase.

f. Give biological source, chemical constituents, and uses of the drug Ergot.

Summer Examination 2001
D Pharm First Year
Pharmacognosy

Q 1. Attempt any *ten* of the following:

a. Define laxatives with two examples.

b. Define pharmacognosy.

c. Write about:
   i. Hippocrates   ii. Sushruta

d. Differentiate between organised and unorganised drugs.

e. Mention the synonyms of:
   i. Aloe   iii. Vinca
   ii. Rhubarb   iv. Cinchona

f. Mention two examples of each of the following used as:
   i. Antitussives   ii. Cardiotonics

g. Mention biological source and family of following crude drugs (any *two*):
   i. Liquorice   iii. Colchicum
   ii. Gymnema

h. Classify following crude drugs according to morphological method of calssification:
  i. Rauwolfia
  ii. Senna
  iii. Aloe
  iv. Cardamom
i. Suggest two drugs for following chemical constituents:
  i. Alkaloids
  ii. Glycosides
  iii. Volatile oils
  iv. Resins
j. What do you know about organoleptic characters of a drug?
k. Mention pharmacological uses of:
  i. Honey
  ii. Vasaka
  iii. Ipecacuanha
  iv. Ergot
l. Name two antirheumatic drugs with sources.

Q 2. Attempt any *three* of the following:

a. Define alkaloids. Classify the alkaloids with examples.
b. Define evaluation. Describe microscopical method of evaluation of crude drug.
c. Describe chemical constituents and uses of digitalis.
d. Draw a well-labelled diagram of TS of fennel or senna.

Q 3. Attempt any *three* of the following:

a. Describe morphological characters of umbelliferous fruits along with diagrams.
b. Describe method of preparation of cotton fibre.
c. Describe pharmacological method of classification of crude drugs.
d. Describe biological source, constituents and uses of ergot.

Q 4. Attempt any *three* of the following:

a. Differentiate sutures and ligatures. Write ideal characters of sutures.
b. Describe the biological source, chemical constituents and uses of drugs containing vitamins.
c. Describe method of collection and preparation of senna.
d. Mention uses of:
  i. Pyrethrum
  ii. Linseed
  iii. Gokharu
  iv. Cinchona

Q 5. Attempt any *three* of the following:

a. Write Keller-Killiani test.
b. Define adulteration. Describe different method of adulteration with suitable examples.
c. Describe general properties of glycosides.

  d. Mention crude drugs for following families.
     i. Apocyanaceae   iii. Leguminosae
     ii. Umbelliferae   iv. Zingiberaceae

Q 6. Explain chemical tests for following crude drugs:
  a. Senna
  b. Rauwolfia
  c. Liquorice
  d. Honey
  e. Opium
  f. Shark liver oil

Winter Examination 2001
D Pharm First Year
Pharmacognosy

Q1. Attempt any *ten* of the following:
  a. Define tannins. Write Gambier fluorescein test for tannins.
  b. Write about:
     i. Aristole   ii. Charak
  c. Define drug.
  d. Define oxytocics and diuretics with examples.
  e. Differentiate plant fibres and animal fibres.
  f. Mention any four drugs for each of the following:
     i. Carminatives   ii. Laxatives
  g. Name examples of crude drugs containing enzymes and vitamins.
  h. Write biological source and uses of:
     i. Ashwagandha   ii. Ginger
  i. Write about different shapes of barks.
  j. Describe external characters of fennel with diagrams.
  k. Mention synonyms of following crude drugs:
     i. Asafoetida   iii. Clove
     ii. Nutmeg   iv. Rauwolfia
  l. Name one antileprotic drug and give its source.

Q 2. Attempt any *three* of the following:
  a. Define evaluation. Describe organoleptic method of evaluation of crude drugs.
  b. Draw well-labelled diagram of TS of cinnamon or datura.
  c. Describe general chemical tests of alkaloids.
  d. Describe chemical constituents of senna or cinchona along with uses.

Q 3. Attempt any *three* of the following:

    a. Describe general methods of collection of barks.

    b. Describe chemical method of classification of crude drugs.

    c. Classify pharmaceutical aid according to their source and mention their uses.

    d. Describe the method of preparation of silk.

Q 4. Attempt any *three* of the following:

    a. Write biological source and uses of:

        i. Beeswax   iii. Shark liver oil

        ii. Dioscorea   iv. Tulsi

    b. Define and classify resins with examples.

    c. Describe method of collection and preparation of Rauwolfia.

    d. Define adulterants and substitutes. Describe various methods of adulteration of crude drugs with suitable examples.

Q 5. Attempt any *three* of the following:

    a. Describe external characters/physical characters of following crude drugs:

        i. Aloe   iii. Gokharu

        ii. Cardamom   iv. Ipecacuanha

    b. Differentiate between roots and rhizomes.

    c. Describe method of isolation of volatile oils.

    d. Describe general properties of tannins.

Q 6. Explain chemical tests of following crude drugs (any *four*):

    a. Aloe

    b. Cinnamon

    c. Ipecacuanha

    d. Starch

    e. Tragacanth

    f. Castor oil

Summer Examination 2002
D Pharm First Year
Pharmacognosy

Q 1. Answer any *five* of the following:

    a. Define pharmacognosy. How this word was coined and who wrote the book 'Analecta Pharmacognostica'?

    b. Explain pharmaceutical aids and classify them giving one example from each class.

c. Give the biological source for (any *two*):
   i. Tobacco iii. Opium
   ii. Lanolin
d. What are terpenoids? Outline in brief their occurrence and distribution in plant.
e. Name which part of the plant is used as a drug in case of following:
   i. Digitalis iii. Gymnema
   ii. Nutmeg iv. Pyrethrum
f. Define with examples (any *two*):
   i. Antirheumatics iii. Antidiabetics
   ii. Laxatives
g. Name the drug which contains:
   i. Emetin iii. Brucine
   ii. Hydnocarpic acid iv. Eugenol

Q 2. Answer any *four* of the following:

a. Explain biological source and diagnostic characters of the drug containing vasicine.
b. What are antiseptics? Give any two examples.
c. Define drug evaluation. Name various methods of drug evaluation.
d. Give biological source, chemical constituents and uses of papaya.
e. Give any two drugs from each of the following families (any *two*):
   i. Scrophulariaceae iii. Leguminosae
   ii. Umbelliferae
f. Explain surgical dressings and sutures.

Q 3.

a. Explain object in classifying crude drug. What are merits and demerits of morphological system of classification of crude drugs?
b. Define alkaloids. How are they classified? Give one example from each class.

Or

Describe microscopic evaluation of crude drugs considering leaf.

Q 4.

a. Describe the histology with a neat and well-labelled diagram of TS of nux-vomica or ipecacuanha and give its uses.
b. Give biological source of silk and explain its preparation.

Q 5. Explain the chemical tests for the following (any *four*):

a. Myrrh d. Ispaghula
b. Black catechu e. Digitalis
c. Aloe f. Turmeric

Q 6.

    a. Name one crude drug uses as (any *four*):

        i. Antitussives   iv. Diuretics

        ii. Adsorbents   v. Vitamins

        iii. Cardiotonics   vi. Emulsifying agents

    b. Describe any *two* of the following:

        i. Describe the general method of isolation of alkaloids.

        ii. Explain, how senna is collected and prepared for te market.

        iii. Differentiate between: Gums and resins.

Winter Examination 2002
D Pharm First Year
Pharmacognosy

Q 1. Answer any *five* of the following:

    a. What is galenical pharmacy? Give contribution of Galen to the pharmacy.

    b. Define flavouring agent: Give any two examples of drugs used as flavouring agents.

    c. Give the biological source for (any *two*):

        i. Lemon grass oil   iii. Beeswax

        ii. Cinchona

    d. What are resins? How are they classified? Give one example from each class.

    e. Name which part of the plant is used as a drug in case of the following:

        i. Vinca   iii. Belladonna

        ii. Arjuna   iv. Cannabis

    f. Define with examples (any *two*):

        i. Carminative   iii. Astringents

        ii. Oxytocics

    g. Name the drug, which contains:

        i. Colchicine   iii. d-linalool

        ii. Vasicine   iv. Kutkoside

Q 2. Answer any *four* of the following:

    a. Explain biological source and diagnostic characters of the drug containing emetine.

    b. What are diuretics? Give any two examples.

    c. Define drug adulteration. Give various methods of drug adulteration with one example from each.

    d. Give biological source, chemical constituents and uses of asafoetida.

    e. Give example of two drugs from each of the following families (any *two*):

        i. Combretaceae   iii. Solanaceae

        ii. Apocyanaceae

    f. What are the official requirements of sutures?

Q 3.

    a. Why crude drugs are classified? Explain advantages and disadvantages of pharmacological system of classification of crude drugs.

    b. Define glycosides. How are they classified? Give one example from each class.

Or

Describe physical method of evaluation of crude drugs considering exhausted drugs.

Q 4.

    a. Describe the histology with a neat and well-labelled diagram of TS of clove or coriander and give its uses.

    b. Explain biological source of cotton. How surgical cotton is prepared?

Q 5. Explain the chemical tests for the following (any *four*):

    a. Honey

    b. Senna

    c. Clove

    d. Agar

    e. Shark liver oil

    f. Pterocarpus

Q 6.

    a. Name one crude drug used as (any *four*):

        i. Carminative

        ii. Laxative

        iii. Enzyme

        iv. Perfumes

        v. Sweetening agent

        vi. Surgical fibre

    b. Answer any two of the following:

        i. Describe the general chemical tests for identification of tannins.

        ii. Explain, how opium is collected and prepared for the market.

        iii. Differentiate between: Volatile oils and fixed oils.

Summer Examination 2003
D Pharm First Year
Pharmacognosy

Q 1. Answer any *ten* of the following:

a. Write about the contribution of following scientists for the development of pharmacognosy.
    i. Seydler   ii. Sushruta

b. Define:
    i. Pharmacognosy   ii. Diuretics

c. Identify following crude drugs with the help of organoleptic evaluation.
    i. Cardamom   ii. Honey

d. Mention the name of crude drug for following chemical constituents:
    i. Emetine   ii. Reserpine

e. Mention biological source of following crude drugs.
    i. Dioscorea   ii. Pyrethrum

f. Write two crude drugs for following families.
    i. Leguminosae   ii. Rubiaceae

g. Write therapeutic uses of:
    i. Guggul   iii. Punarnava
    ii. Chaulmoogra oil   iv. Cinchona

h. Describe external morphological characters with the help of sketches of:
    i. Aconite   ii. Gokharu

i. Describe any two methods of extracting volatile oils.

j. Classify following crude drugs with the help of morphological method of classification of crude drugs.
    i. Nux-vomica   iii. Ipecac
    ii. Opium   iv. Cinchona

k. Write chemical test of liquorice and ipecac.

Q 2. Answer any *two* of the following:

a. Define alkaloids. Describe properties of alkaloids. Classify the alkaloids.

b. Define pharmaceutical aids. Classify pharmaceutical aids along with their uses.

c. Describe cultivation and collection of digitalis.

Q 3. Answer any *two* of the following:

a. Draw well-labelled diagram of TS of fennel fruit. Describe microscopical characters of fennel fruit.

    b. Define drug evaluation. Write different methods of drug evaluation. Describe biological method of drug evaluation.

    c. Describe different methods of classification of crude drugs.

Q 4. Answer any *three* of the following:

    a. Describe method of preparation of silk fibre.

    b. Write water soluble and water insoluble pairs of ergot alkaloids.

    c. Describe biological source, chemical constituents and uses of:

        i. Lanolin   ii. Shatavari

    d. Draw well-labelled diagram showing external parts of:

        i. Nux-vomica   ii. Clove

Q 5. Answer any *three* of the following:

    a. Define laxatives. Describe biological source, chemical constituents, and uses of aloes.

    b. Define carminatives. Describe with sketches the external characters of nutmeg.

    c. Describe the uses of:

        i. Neem   ii. Liquorice

    d. Write the synonyms of:

        i. Ephedra   iii. Vasaka

        ii. Aconite   iv. Vinca

Q 6. Describe chemical tests of following crude drug.

    a. Senna   d. Cinchona

    b. Pale catechu   e. Honey

    c. Shark liver oil   f. Turmeric

Winter Examination 2003
D Pharm First Year
Pharmacognosy

Q 1. Answer any *five* of the following:

    a. Differentiate plant fibre and animal fibre.

    b. Define:

        i. Oxytocics   ii. Synonyms

    c. Draw well-labelled diagram showing external morphological parts of:

        i. Fennel   ii. Isapaghula seed

    d. Give the name of the crude drug containing following chemical constituents.

        i. Oxidase   ii. Bassorine

e. Give synonyms of following crude drugs.
   i. Ginger
   ii. Opium
f. Give one example of crude drug which is having following pharmacological action.
   i. Carminative
   ii. Antispasmodic
g. Define "emollient" with two examples of crude drugs.
h. Mention crude drug which shows following microscopical characters (draw sketches):
   i. Paracytic stomata
   ii. Anisocytic stomata
i. What do you know about:
   i. Papyrus ebers   ii. Galen
j. Describe chemical tests for following crude drugs.
   i. Rauwolfia   ii. Starch

Q 2. Answer any *two* of the following:

a. Describe life cycle of ergot along with diagrams.
b. Define glycosides. Mention method of isolation of glycosides.
c. Define drug evaluation. Describe organoleptic method of drug evaluation.

Q 3. Answer any *two* of the following:

a. Draw well-labelled diagram of TS of coriander fruit. Describe microscopy of coriander fruit.
b. Describe any two methods of classification of crude drugs. Mention the classification of laxatives alongwith examples of crude drugs.
c. Describe method of preparation of wool fibre.

Q 4. Answer any *three* of the following:

a. What is the importance of perfumes and flavouring agents? Describe biological source and chemical constituents of lemon grass oil and sandal wood oil.
b. Mention biological source and family of:
   i. Vinca   ii. Benzoin
c. Describe therapeutic uses of:
   i. Digitalis   iii. Pterocarpus
   ii. Senna   iv. Gokharu
d. Which parts or form of the following crude drugs are used as a drug:
   i. Senna   iii. Tulsi
   ii. Opium   iv. Vinca

Q 5. Answer any three of the following:

  a. Mention crude drugs for following families:

      i. Zygophyllaceae   iii. Zingiberaceae

      ii. Scrophulariaceae   iv. Umbelliferous

  b. Describe chemical constituents of digitalis and aloes.

  c. Mention two crude drugs for rach containing resins and tannins.

  d. Define adulteration. Describe any one method of adulteration of crude drugs.

Q 6. Describe chemical tests of following crude drugs (any _four_):

  a. Digitalis   d. Benzoin

  b. Castor oil   e. Linseed

  c. Asafoetida   f. Gelatin

Summer Examination 2004
D Pharm First Year
Pharmacognosy

Q 1. Attempt any _ten_ of the following:

  a. Define crude drug.

  b. How the 'pharmacognosy' word coined and who coined it?

  c. Write about:

      i. Hippocrates   ii. Aristotle

  d. Explain Kellar-Killiani test for digitalis.

  e. Define balsam. How will you detect true balsams.

  f. Which part of the plant is used as drug in case of:

      i. Gymnema   iii. Rhubarb

      ii. Vinca   iv. Cannabis

  g. Define with examples (any _two_):

      i. Astringents   iii. Antirheumatics

      ii. Antiseptics

  h. Name the drug which contains:

      i. Brucine   iii. Vitamin A

      ii. Morphine   iv. Quinine

  i. Describe external characters of gokharu with diagrams.

  j. Differentiate between plant fibre and animal fibre.

  k. Write biological source and uses of:

      i. Arjuna   iii. Pterocarpus

      ii. Lemon grass oil   iv. Ephedra

Q 2. Attempt any *three* of the following:

  a. Draw well-labelled diagram of TS of cinchona bark or clove bud.

  b. Define drug evaluation. Describe chemical method of drug evaluation.

  c. Define and classify terpenoids with examples.

  d. Describe method of collection and preparation of senna for market.

Q 3. Attempt any *three* of the following:

  a. Describe morphological method of classification of crude drugs with its merit and demerits.

  b. What is adulteration? Give various methods with suitable examples.

  c. Define alkaloids. Give any two general chemical tests for identification of alkaloids.

  d. Give chemical constituents and uses of (any *two*):

     i. Ginger   iii. Picrorrhiza

     ii. Amla   iv. Agar

Q 4. Attempt any *three* of the following:

  a. Describe the method of preparation of silk.

  b. Give any two examples of drug from each of the following families (any *two*):

     i. Umbelliferae

     ii. Solanaceae

     iii. Combretaceae

  c. Define resins. How are they classified?

  d. How will you differentiate:

     i. Acacia and tragacanth

     ii. Volatile oil and fixed oil

Q 5. Attempt any *three* of the following:

  a. What are the official requirements of sutures.

  b. Name the drug used as insecticide. Give its biological source, chemical constituents and uses.

  c. What are cardiotonics? Give any two exmaples.

  d. Give biological source, chemical constituents and uses of black catechu.

Q 6. Explain chemical tests of following crude drugs (any *four*):

  a. Benzoin   e. Honey

  b. Clove   f. Nux-vomica

  c. Arachis oil

  d. Digitalis

Summer Examination 2005
D Pharm First Year
Pharmacognosy

Q 1. Attempt any *ten* of the following:

   a. Define diuretics with examples.

   b. Explain "Borntrager's test" for senna.

   c. Which parts of the plant is used as a drug in case of:

      i. Nux-vomica   iii. Arjuna

      ii. Ginger   iv. Gokharu

   d. Differentiate between leaf and leaflet.

   e. Classify the pharmaceutical aids according to their sources.

   f. Write biological source and uses of:

      i. Pterocarpus   ii. Ephedra

   g. Explain the role of "Dioscorides" and "Galen" in the development of pharmacognosy.

   h. Name the drugs which contains:

      i. Emetine   iii. Arabin

      ii. Aconitine   iv. Colchicine

   i. Mention synonyms of following crude drugs.

      i. Tulsi   iii. Rhubarb

      ii. Aconite   iv. Pyrethrum

   j. Describe external characters of nutmeg with diagrams.

   k. Define crude drugs.

   l. Name the crude drugs acting on nervous system.

Q 2. Attempt any *three* of the following:

   a. Describe the chemical method of classification of crude drugs with its merits and demerits.

   b. Define volatile oil and classify them.

   c. What are "cardiotonics"? Give biological source and chemical constituents of any one.

   d. Explain the "organoleptic" method for evaluation of crude drugs.

   e. Explain in short "indigenous system of medicine".

Q 3. Attempt any *three* of the following:

   a. Define resins. How are they classified?

   b. Give biological source, chemical constituents and uses of Ashwagandha.

   c. Describe the method for preparation of absorbent cotton.

   d. Draw well-labelled diagram of TS of nux vomica.

   e. Give chemical constituents and uses of fennel.

Q 4. Attempt any *three* of the following:
  a. How will you differentiate?
      i. Organised and unorganized crude drugs.
      ii. Roots and rhizomes.
  b. Give the chemical constituents and uses of:
      i. Opium   ii. Ergot
  c. Name the adulterants and substituents of (any *two*):
      i. Rauwolfia
      ii. Nux-vomica
      iii. Digitalis
  d. Explain the diagnostic features of aconite.
  e. Indian dill is not suitable for human use. Why?

Q 5. Attempt any *three* of the following:
  a. Define and classify glycosides.
  b. Define antitussives. Give biological source and chemical constituents of any one.
  c. Give chemical constituents and uses of (any *two*):
      i. Gymnema   iii. Amla
      ii. Clove   iv. Sandal wood
  d. Define and classify tannins with examples.
  e. Give biological source and family of black catechu.

Q 6. Explain chemical tests of following crude drugs (any *four*):
  a. Clove   d. Ipecacuanha
  b. Asafoetida   e. Opium
  c. Myrrh   f. Acacia

Winter Examination 2005
D Pharm First Year
Pharmacognosy

Q 1. Attempt any *ten* of the following:
  a. Mention synonyms of the following crude drugs.
      i. Nutmeg   iii. Agar
      ii. Rauwolfia   iv. Ginger
  b. Write biological source and uses of:
      i. Chaulmoogra   ii. Pterocarpus
  c. Differentiate between surgical suture and ligature.
  d. Describe the external characters of cinchona with diagram.

e. Name the crude drug which contains:
   i. D-linalool   iii. Vincristine
   ii. Myricin   iv. Linamarine
f. Define with examples:
   i. Astringents   iii. Diuretics
   ii. Antitussives
g. Which part of the plant is used as a drug in case of:
   i. Clove   iii. Guggul
   ii. Aconite   iv. Gelatin
h. Define fibre. Name three animal fibres.
i. Explain combined umbelliferone test for asafoetida.
j. What is charak samhita and shushrut samhita?
k. Name three crude drugs from mineral source.
l. Define pharmacognosy.
m. Define pharmaceutical aids with examples.
n. Give any four official requirements regarding surgical dressings.

Q 2. Attempt any *three* of the following:

a. Describe the process of drying of crude drugs.
b. Name the drug used as oxytocic. Give its biological source, chemical constituents and uses.
c. What are laxatives? Give any three examples.
d. Give the biological source, chemical constituents and uses of garlic.

Q 3. Attempt any *three* of the following:

a. Describe the method of preparation of absorbent cotton.
b. Give any two examples of crude drugs from each of the following families (any *two*):
   i. Apocynaceae   iii. Scrophalariaceae
   ii. Leguminoceae
c. Define glycosides. How are they classified on the basis of chemical nature of aglycone?
d. How will you differentiate:
   i. Sumatra benzoin and siam benzoin
   ii. Fats and waxes
e. Explain the term entire organism with examples.

Q 4. Attempt any *three* of the following:

a. Describe pharmacological method of classification of crude drugs with suitable examples.
b. What is adulteration? Give various methods of adulteration with suitable examples.

c. Define tannins. Give any two general chemical tests for identification of tannins.

d. Give chemical constituents and uses of (any *two*):
  i. Fennel   iii. Dioscorea
  ii. Ephedra   iv. Neem

e. Give biological source and uses of 'sandal wood'.

Q 5. Attempt any *three* of the following:

a. Draw a well-labelled diagram of TS of cinnamon bark.

b. Define evaluation. Describe microscopic method of evaluation of crude drugs.

c. Define and classify alkaloids with examples.

d. Describe the method of collection and preparation of digitalis for the market.

e. Define the terms:
  i. Crude drug   ii. Carminative

Q 6. Explain the chemical test of the following crude drugs (any *four*):

a. Senna
b. Ipecacunha
c. Nux vomica
d. Curcuma
e. Shark liver oil
f. Starch

Summer Examination 2006
D Pharm First Year
Pharmacognosy

Q 1. Attempt any *ten* of the following:

a. Mention synonyms of the following crude drugs.
  i. Rauwolfia   iii. Nux vomica
  ii. Gokharu   iv. Ajiwan

b. Write the biological source of:
  i. Aloe   ii. Vinca

c. Define fibres. Give the examples of plant fibres along with the biological source of cotton.

d. Give the identification test for starch.

e. Differentiate between perfumes and flavouring agents along with the examples of each.

f. Define stomatal index. How it can be calculated?

g. State the different underground modifications of stem with their examples.

h. Define pharmacognosy.

i. What is morphological classification of crude drugs?

j. Write the contribution of following scientists in history of pharmacognosy.

    i. Galen

    ii. Dioscorides

    iii. Hippocrates

    iv. Charak

k. Define resin. Give different resin combination along with examples.

l. Define surgical sutures. Which are the properties they must possess?

m. Define with examples.

    i. Febrifugal

    ii. Stomachic

n. Define pesticides. Give two examples of pesticide along with the biological source for any one of it.

Q 2. Attempt any *three* of the following:

a. Explain the term cardiotonics and state the biological source of digitalis along with its chemical constituents.

b. Define crude drug. Who has coined the word pharmacognosy. How it was coined?

c. Define with one example.

    i. Dried juices

    ii. Latex

    iii. Balsams

    iv. Extracts

d. What is adulteration? State different means of adulterating crude drugs.

e. What are volatile oils? State the different techniques for isolation of volatile oils.

Q 3. Attempt any *three* of the following:

a. What are laxatives? Give two examples of laxative drugs. What is biological source and chemical constituents of isapgol seed.

b. What is pharmacological classification and chemical classification of natural drugs?

c. Differentiate between organized and unorganized crude drug.

d. What are alkaloids? What are different identification tests for alkaloids?

e. Give biological source and transverse section and pharmacognostic features of fennel.

Q 4. Attempt any *three* of the following:

a. What are astringents? What is the difference between black catechu and pale catechu.

b. Give the test for identification, adulterants and substituents of nux-vomica seed.

c. Define antitussives with examples. Give biological source, chemical constituents and uses of vasaka.

d. What are pharmaceutical aids. Give different sources for it along with the classification.

e. What are antimalarials? Give the chemical constituents, biological source of cinchona bark?

Q 5. Attempt any *three* of the following:

a. What are oxytocics? Give the life cycle of ergot.

b. What are traditional systems of medicine? Give examples of Ayurvedic and Herbal formulations in market.

c. State the borntrager test. Give the chemical constituents and uses of senna leaf.

d. What are enzymes? What is the biological source, chemical constituents and uses of papaya?

e. Draw a well-labelled diagram of TS of senna leaf. What is the difference between upper and lower palisade cells of senna?

Q 6. Attempt any *three* of the following:

a. What are vitamins? Give the biological source, chemical constituents and uses of amla fruit?

b. Explain the chemical test for (any *two*):
   i. Turmeric
   ii. Honey
   iii. Acacia

c. Give the examples of drugs that are obtained from animal source with the biological source, chemical constituents and uses of any one of it.

d. Define antiseptics and disinfectants. Write the biological source and uses of neem and benzoin.

e. Define with examples.
   i. Antileprotics
   ii. Diuretics
   iii. Antidiabetics
   iv. Carminatives

Winter Examination 2006
D Pharm First Year
Pharmacognosy

Q 1. Answer any *ten* of the following:

a. Define:
    i. Crude drug   ii. Adulteration
b. How is Indian senna collected and prepared for the market.
c. What do you know about "siddha system of medicine?
d. Give the geographical distribution of curcuma.
e. What enhances the use of morphological classification of crude drugs?
f. Mention a crude drug for which each of the following synonym is applicable.
    i. Jayphal   iii. Sarpgandha
    ii. Puncture vine   iv. Adulsa
g. What is the significance of following chemical tests when agar is treated with:
    i. Ruthenium red solution
    ii. Fehling's solution and boiled
h. Who was shushruta? Describe his contribution in the development of pharmacognosy.
i. Which chemical class is identified by modified Borntrager's test? How will you perform it?
j. Which is the recent method of classification of crude drugs? Describe it with one examples.
k. Mention which part of the plant is useful as a drug in case of:
    i. Clove   iii. Aconite
    ii. Vasaka   iv. Arjuna
l. What is the significance of acid-insoluble ash in evaluation of crude drugs? Explain with a suitable example.
m. Describe Ecuelle process of expression of volatile oils. Name a volatile oil isolated by this process.
n. A surface preparation of an upper epidermis of a leaf shows 5 stomata/sq. mm and 20 epidermal cells in the same unit area. Calculate stomatal index of the said leaf surface.

Q 2. Answer any *three* of the following:

a. Differentiate between hydrolysable tannins and condensed tannins.
b. Give the classification of volatile oils with examples.
c. Describe a method of isolation of glycosides from the crude drugs.

d. Describe contribution of following persons in the development of pharmacognosy.
    i. CA Seydler   ii. Hippocrates
e. Where will you classify the drugs digitalis, ipecacuanha, cinnamon and amla each in:
    i. Morphological classification
    ii. Pharmacological classification

Q 3. Answer any *three* of the following:

a. Describe a method of preparation of an animal fibre containing a protein 'keratin'.
b. Write morphological characters with diagram of a fruit drug of family piperaceae.
c. Draw a well-labelled diagram of a TS of a crude drug of family myrtaceae especially labelling the tissues containing:
    i. Voltaile oil
    ii. Air spaces
d. Describe taxonomical classification of crude drugs with one example and its demerits.
e. Write chemical constituents and uses of a fruit drug from family zingiberaceae.

Q 4. Answer any *three* of the following:

a. Write two synonyms for each of the following:
    i. Cinchona
    ii. Arachis oil
b. Write two chemical tests for identification of shark liver oil.
c. What do you mean by "bio-assay"? Describe it briefly giving names of two crude drugs that can be subjected to bio-assay.
d. Give occurrence and distribution of alkaloids in nature.
e. Define with two examples:
    i. Pharmaceutical aids
    ii. Diuretics
f. Write biological source of:
    i. Lanolin   ii. Linseed

Q 5. Answer any *three* of the following:

a. Give two examples each of crude drug containing
    i. Anthraquinone glycosides   iii. Oleogum resin
    ii. Tropane alkaloids   iv. Starch
b. How will you distinguish pale catechu from black catechu using different chemical tests.
c. Write source, chemical nature and uses of kaolin.

    d. Give two examples each of crude drug from family.

        i. Liliaceae   iii. Euphorbiaceae

        ii. Apocyanaceae   iv. Scrophulariaceae

    e. Name different titles under which any drug is studied systematically in pharmacognosy.

Q 6. Answer any *three* of the following:

    a.   i. Name a crude drug to which each of the following chemical test is applicable.

            1. Test for meconic acid   3. Keller-Killani test

            2. Fiche's test   4. Vitali-Morin test

        ii. How crude drugs are adulterated by replacement by exhausted drugs?

    b. Describe utility of following in microscopic evaluation of crude drugs.

        i. Phloem fibre   ii. Palisade ratio

    c.   i. Draw well-labelled diagrams of Isapgol seed as seen from dorsal and ventral surface.

        ii. Write the uses of silk.

    d. Write two tests that distinguish gum acacia from Tragacanth.

    e. Write any four therapeutic effects of glycosides with one example of crude drug for each effect.

Summer Examination 2007
D Pharm First Year
Pharmacognosy

Q 1. Answer any *ten* of the following:

    a. Define pharmacognosy. Write contribution of Charak and Galen in development of pharmacognosy.

    b. Name the drugs which contain:

        i. Vincristine   iii. Scopolamine

        ii. Reserpine   iv. Piperine

    c. Write chemical constituents and uses of:

        i. Rauwolfia   ii. Vinca

    d. Define Tannins. Write chemical tests for tannins.

    e. Define antitussives with examples. Give biological source, chemical constituents of vasaka.

    f. Draw a well-labelled diagram showing external morphological characters of:

        i. Fennel   ii. Ispaghula seed

g. What are enzymes? Give biological source and chemical constituents of papaya.

h. Define and classify pharmaceutical aids, according to their uses.

i. Define fibres. Give examples of animal fibres along with biological source and chemical constituents of silk.

j. Write biological source and uses of:
   i. Cinnamon bark
   ii. Gymnema

k. Name drug uses as antidysentric. Give biological source and chemical constituent for same.

l. Explain 'Borntrager's test' for senna.

m. Mention synonyms of following drugs:
   i. Ephedra
   ii. Clove
   iii. Ashwagandha
   iv. Nutmeg

n. Define surgical dressing. What are ideal requirements for surgical dressings?

Q 2. Attempt any *three* of the following:

a. Explain "Drying" in preparation of crude drug for market.

b. How will you differentiate:
   i. Organized and unorganized drug
   ii. Gums and resins

c. Describe pharmacological method of classification with its merits and demerits.

d. What are vitamins? Give biological source, chemical constituents and uses of Amla.

e. Define Adulteration. Give various methods of adulteration with suitable examples.

Q 3. Attempt any *three* of the following:

a. What are volatile oils? State different techniques for isolation of volatile oils.

b. Explain 'Microscopic method' for evaluation of crude drug?

c. Write synonym, biological source, chemical constituent, uses, adulterants and substituents of nux vomica.

d. Define and classify resin. Give different resin combination along with example.

e. Draw well-labelled diagram of TS of cinchona bark. Describe its microscopy.

Q 4. Attempt any *three* of the following:

   a. Define oxytocics. Describe life cycle of Ergot along with diagram.

   b. Describe cultivation, collection, preparation for market of digitalis.

   c. Describe antiseptic and disinfectant. Give biological source, chemical constituents of turmeric and neem.

   d. Describe method of preparation of silk fibre.

   e. What is the importance of perfumes and flavouring agents. Write biological source, and chemical constituents of peppermint oil and lemon oil.

Q 5. Attempt any *three* of the following:

   a. What are glycosides? Explain Keller-Killani test for cardiac glycosides?

   b. Explain chemical tests for (any *two*):
     i. Starch
     ii. Agar
     iii. Acacia

   c. Define antileprotic. Give biological source, chemical constituents of chaulmoogra oil.

   d. Write biological source and uses of:
     i. Garlic
     ii. Shankhpushpi
     iii. Glycerrhiza
     iv. Shatavari

   e. Define with examples.
     i. Diuretics
     ii. Antirheumatics
     iii. Astringents
     iv. Carminatives

Q 6. Attempt any *three* of the following:

   a. Define with one example:
     i. Dried juices
     ii. Latex
     iii. Gum and mucilages
     iv. Extracts

   b. Define alkaloids. Give chemical tests for identification of alkaloids by precipitation method.

   c. Write about 'Ayurveda' and Traditional Indian system of medicines'.

   d. Define laxatives. Draw well-labelled diagram of TS of senna leaf.

   e. Define cardiotonics. Write biological source, chemical constituents, adulterant and substituents of digitalis.

Winter Examination 2007
D Pharm First Year
Pharmacognosy

Q 1. Answer any *ten* of the following:

a. Define pharmacognosy. Who coin the word pharmacognosy?

b. Write about

    i. Ayurveda   ii. Hippocrates

c. Match the following:

    i. Gum   a. Opium

    ii. Juice   b. Acacia

    iii. Extract   c. Aloe

    iv. Latex   d. Gelatin

d. Which part of the plant is used as a drug in case of:

    i. Vasaka   iii. Ginger

    ii. Shatavari   iv. Ephedra

e. Define with examples.

    i. Carminatives   ii. Diuretics

f. Name the drug which contain

    i. Vitamin A   iii. Linamarin

    ii. Emetine   iv. Allicine

g. Explain 'Gold beater skin test' for tannins.

h. Mention the synonyms of following crude drugs.

    i. Vinca   iii. Cinnamon

    ii. Lanolin   iv. Gokharu

i. Write the biological source of:

    i. Arachis oil   iii. Amla

    ii. Arjuna   iv. Ashwagandha

Q 2. Answer any *three* of the following:

a. Differentiate between organized and unorganized crude drugs with examples.

b. Describe pharmacological method of classification of crude drugs with its merits and demerits.

c. Define drug adulteration. Mention different methods of drug adulteration with examples.

d. Draw well-labelled diagram of TS of nux vomica and describe the same.

e. Define alkaloids. Explain general chemical tests of alkaloids.

Q 3. Answer any *three* of the following:

   a. Define drug evaluation. Explain why moisture content is important for evaluation of crude drugs with examples.

   b. What are glycosides? How they are isolated from plant?

   c. Describe method of cultivation, collection and preparation of Rauwolfia for market.

   d. Define and classify volatile oils with suitable examples.

   e. Give the biological source, chemical constituents and uses of senna.

Q 4. Answer any *three* of the following:

   a. Define pharmaceutical aids. Classify according to their use and application with suitable examples.

   b. Mention the adulterants of honey and explain the chemical test for detection of adulterants.

   c. What are astringents? Give the biological source, chemical constituents and uses of black catechu.

   d. Describe the method of preparation of silk fibre.

   e. Name two examples of crude drugs from each of the following families.

      i. Labiatae   iii. Bruseraceae

      ii. Rubiaceae   iv. Rutaceae

Q 5. Answer any *three* of the following:

   a. Define sutures. What are the ideal requirements of sutures?

   b. What are cardiotonics? Give biological source, chemical constituents and uses of any one.

   c. Mention adulterants of clove and substitutes of nutmeg.

   d. Name the drug having following chemical test and explain any one of them.

      i. Modified Borntrager test

      ii. Guignard test

      iii. Keller-Killani test

      iv. Vitali-Morin test

   e. Define and classify resins with examples.

Q 6. Explain chemical tests of following crude drugs.

   a. Agar

   b. Clove

   c. Asafoetida

   d. Turmeric

   e. Nux vomica

   f. Wool

Summer Examination 2008
D Pharm First Year
Pharmacognosy

Q 1. Answer any *ten* of the following:

a. Define with examples.
    i. Antiseptics   iii. Oxytocics
    ii. Astringents

b. Define crude drugs. Give three examples of crude drugs from mineral source.

c. Explain combined Umbelliferone test for asafoetida.

d. Write about:
    i. Hippocrates   ii. Dioscorides

e. Mention four characters of umbelliferous fruit.

f. Define terpenoids. What are the uses of terpenoids.

g. Name the crude drug which contains:
    i. Aldobionic acid   iii. Kino red
    ii. Fenchone   iv. Emetine

h. Which part of the plant is used as drug in case of:
    i. Aloe   iii. Ginger
    ii. Clove   iv. Senna

i. Differentiate between fats and waxes.

j. Describe external characters of coriander with diagram.

k. Mention synonyms of following crude drugs.
    i. Nutmeg   iii. Tulsi
    ii. Ephedra   iv. Gokharu

l. Write biological source and uses of:
    i. Colchicum   ii. Vinca

Q 2. Answer any *three* of the following:

a. Name one drug used as antihypertensive, give its biological source, chemical constituents and uses.

b. What are volatile oils? How are they classified?

c. Describe the life cycle and collection of ergot for the market.

d. How will you differentiate between.
    i. Gums and resins   ii. Volatile oil and fixed oil

Q 3. Answer any *three* of the following:

a. Define alkaloids. Describe the properties of alkaloids.

b. Give chemical constituents and uses of (any *two*):
    i. Senna   iii. Ergot
    ii. Ashwagandha   iv. Pyrethrum

c. Describe morphological method of classification of crude drugs with its merits and demerits.

d. Define adulteration. Give various methods of adulteration with suitable examples.

Q 4. Answer any *three* of the following:

a. Describe method of collection and preparation of digitalis for the market.

b. Name the different methods of drug evaluation. Describe any *four* microscopic method of evaluation of crude drugs.

c. Draw a neat labelled diagram of TS of fennel and describe the same.

d. Define perfumes and flavouring agents. Give the biological source, family, chemical constituents and uses of any *two*.

Q 5. Answer any *three* of the following:

a. Describe pharmaceutical aids with examples.

b. Give two examples of drugs from each of the following families (any *two*).

    i. Zingiberaceae   iii. Solanaceae

    ii. Euphorbiaceae

c. Describe the method of preparation of silk.

d. Give biological source, chemical constituents and uses of cinnamon bark.

Q 6. Explain chemical tests of following crude drugs which contains following active chemical constituents (any *four*).

a. Quinine   d. Vitamin A

b. Cephalin   e. Agarose

c. Sennoside A and B   f. Natural invert sugar

Winter Examination 2008
D Pharm First Year
Pharmacognosy

Q 1. Answer any *five* of the following:

a. Define 'pharmacognosy'. When , where and who coined the term 'pharmacognosy'?

b. Which crude drug is represented by each of the following?

    i. *Evolvulus alsinoides*   iii. *Claviceps purpurea*

    ii. Cera flava   iv. Oleum selachoide

c. Name a cardiotonic leaf drug studied by you. How is it collected and prepared for the market?

d. What do you mean by pharmacopoeial standards? Name its types. Describe significance of 'Total Ash Content' with an example.

e. Give two examples of crude drugs from each family:
   i. Solanaceae   iii. Rubiaceae
   ii. Zingiberaceae   iv. Labiatae

f. Differentiate between organised crude drugs and unorganised crude drugs with examples.

g. Define with *two* examples of each.
   i. Dried juices   ii. Antitussive

Q 2. Answer any *three* of the following:

a. Describe contribution of following persons in development of pharmacognosy.
   i. Charak   ii. Dioscorides

b. Explain the terms charas, hashish, ganja and write its biological source.

c. Name a crude drug that fits for each of the following statement.
   i. A mineral substance used as an adsorbent.
   ii. An antioxytoxic, galactagogue drug of family Liliaceae
   iii. A protein extract from animal bones, tendons and skin
   iv. Native of Myanmar, Thailand, Eastern parts of India, Indonesia is used in the treatment of TB and Leprosy.

d. Describe methods for isolation of volatile oils from the crude drugs.

e. What do you mean by the word 'Organoleptic'? Describe organoleptic evaluation of crude drugs with suitable examples.

Q 3. Answer any *three* of the following:

a. Give classification of glycosides with examples of each crude drug.

b. i. Define an 'Adulterant'. Correlate any two reasons/conditions with adulteration of crude drugs.
   ii. Name the method of adulteration used in case of:
      1. Artificial invert sugar is mixed with honey
      2. A person collects rhubarb rhizomes from 5 years old plant and adds to genuine drug.

c. Describe 'Ayurveda' as indigenous system of medicine.

d. Write biological source of:
   i. Nutmeg   ii. Asafoetida

e. i. Write two chemical tests for identification of nux-vomica.
   ii. Write two synonyms for each
      1. Rauwolfia   2. Honey

Q 4. Answer any *three* of the following:

a. Describe pharmacological classification of crude drugs with examples from two different categories. State its one disadvantage.

b. Which umbelliferous fruit mainly contains a chemical compound linalol? Write its morphological characters with diagram.

c. Write chemical constituents and uses of a flower bud of family myrtacear.

d. Draw a well labelled cellular diagram of a TS of a bark drug used as antimalarial or carminative.

e. Describe a method of preparation of a plant fibre from your syllabus.

Q 5. Answer any *three* of the following:

a. Write biological source, chemical constituents and uses of Lanolin.

b. Give two examples each of crude drug containing:
   i. Vitamins   iii. Mucilage
   ii. Indole alkaloids   iv. Tannins

c. How will you distinguish silk fibres from wool fibres using different solubility tests, chemical tests and microscopic examination?

d. Explain the significance of following in evaluation of crude drugs with suitable examples:
   i. Optical rotation   ii. Ether soluble extractives

e. Give occurrence and distribution of alkaloids in nature.

Q 6. Answer any *three* of the following:

a. i. Mention which part of the plant is useful as a drug in case of:
      1. Gymnema   3. Arjuna
      2. Black pepper   4. Aconite

   ii. How crude drugs are adulterated by 'Addition of other parts of the same plant'? Give two examples.

b. Define 'Resins' with one example from animal source. Give two examples of crude drugs containing resins that have each of the following therapeutic effect:
   i. Expectorant   ii. Carminative

c. i. Write uses of wood.

   ii. Give geographical distribution of cinnamon.

d. i. Draw a well-labelled diagram of Ephedra.

   ii. Name four crude drugs used as laxatives.

e. i. For identification of which crude drugs 'Swelling Factor' is determined. Describe how will you determine it?

   ii. Name a crude drug containing:
      1. Kutkin   3. Bassorin
      2. Barbaloin   4. Morphine

Summer Examination 2009
D Pharm First Year
Pharmacognosy

Q 1. Answer any *eight* of the following:

a. When, where and who coined the term 'Pharmacognosy'?

b. Name any five indigenous systems of medicine.

c. What enhances the use of alphabetical classification of crude drugs?

d. What do you mean by pharmacopoeial standards? Name its types.

e. How is ergot collected and prepared for the market?

f. Name three sources of fibres with an example from any two sources.

g. Define the term 'Laxatives' with three examples.

h. Who is known as 'Father of Medicine'? Describe his contribution in development of Pharmacognosy.

i. Define 'Alkaloids' and name any two alkaloids.

j. State any five reasons or conditions for adulteration of crude drugs.

k. What is the significance of 'Keller-Killiani Test'? Explain how it is performed?

l. Define 'Pharmaceutical Aids' with its any three types.

Q 2. Answer any *three* of the following:

a. Which umbelliferous fruit contains 'linalool' as a major chemical compound? Write its morphological characters with a labelled diagram.

b. Write biological source of:
  i. Acacia   ii. Nutmeg

c. Draw a well-labelled cellular diagram of a TS of a bark drug used as antimalarial. Show also the tissues containing starch and calcium oxalate crystals in it.

d. Write chemical constituents and uses of clove.

e. Describe pharmacological classification of crude drugs with examples from two different categories. State its one disadvantages.

Q 3. Answer any *three* of the following:

a. Differentiate between organised and unorganised crude drugs with examples.

b. Give occurrence and distribution of volatile oils in nature.

c. i. Name a crude drug containing:
  1. Fenchone   3. Curcumin
  2. Oleo-gum-resin   4. Bassorin

    ii. How crude drugs are adulterated by 'Addition of other parts of the same plant'? Give two examples.

d. i. Write uses of Absorbent Cotton.

    ii. Name any four classes (types) of glycosides.

e. i. Mention which part of the plant is useful as a drug in case of:

    1. Aconite   3. Gymnema

    2. Gokhru   4. Arjuna

    ii. What do you mean by 'Swelling Factor'? What is its significance? Describe how you will determine it?

Q 4. Answer any *three* of the following:

a. i. Why is Borntrager's test modified for Aloe? Describe how it is performed?

    ii. Write any four therapeutic uses of tannins with suitable examples.

b. Describe the ancient Indian system of medicine.

c. i. Write two synonyms for each

    1. Rauwolfia   2. Honey

    ii. Write two chemicals tests for indentification of nux-vomica.

d. Describe a method of preparation of wool fibres.

e. i. Which chemical substance is responsible for pungent taste of:

    1. Black pepper   2. Ginger

    ii. State the choice of an evaluation method you will use for

    1. Confirming identity of a leaf drug

    2. Determining anticancer activity of a new drug.

Q 5. Answer any *three* of the following:

a. Describe contribution of following persons in development of pharmacognosy.

    i. Sushruta

    ii. Galen

b. Where will you classify the crude drugs Cardamom, Senna, Opium and Benzoin each in:

    i. Taxonomical classification? (Name only family)

    ii. Chemical classification

c. Describe a method for isolation of alkaloids from the crude drug.

d. What do you mean by 'Organoleptic Evaluation'? Describe it with suitable examples of crude drugs.

e. Differentiate between condensed tannins and hydrolysable tannins.

Q 6. Answer any *three* of the following:

a. Give two examples each of the crude drug containing
   - i. Indole alkaloids
   - ii. Enzymes
   - iii. Mucilage
   - iv. Vitamins

b. Write biological source, chemical constituents and uses of Lanolin.

c. How will you distinguish silk fibres from wool fibres using different solubility tests, chemical tests and microscopic examination?

d. Give two examples of crude drugs from each family:
   - i. Rubiaceae
   - ii. Solanaceae
   - iii. Liliaceae
   - iv. Euphorbiaceae

e. Explain the significance of following in evaluation of crude drugs with suitable examples:
   - i. Water soluble extractives
   - ii. Optical rotation

Summer Examination 2010
D Pharm First Year
Pharmacognosy

Q 1. Attempt any *ten* of the following:

a. Define pharmacognosy.

b. Write about contribution of following scientist for development of pharmacognosy:
   - i. Seydler
   - ii. Charak.

c. Write synonyms of following crude drugs:
   - i. Aloes
   - ii. Gokhru
   - iii. Vasaka
   - iv. Honey

d. Define oxytocic and expectorant with example.

e. Give the example of:
   - i. Emetic
   - ii. Antisepic

f. Write one crude drug from each family:
   - i. Apocynaceae
   - ii. Leguminosae
   - iii. Burseraceae
   - iv. Zygophyllaceae.

g. Mention crude drug which shows following characters:
   - i. Parquetry arrangement of cells.
   - ii. Paracytic stomata.

h. Differentiate between organized and unorganized crude drugs.

i. Draw well labelled diagrams showing external morphological characters of Fennel.

j. Write uses of:
   - i. Kaolin
   - ii. Papaya

k. Name the crude drug which contain:
   i. Ricinoleic acid   ii. Mucilage
   iii. Piperine   iv. Reserpine
l. Define pharmaceutical aids with two examples.

Q 2. Attempt any *three* of the following:

a. Describe life cycle of Ergot alongwith diagrams.
b. Define glycosides. Classify glycosides with examples.
c. Define evaluation of crude drugs. Describe any three microscopical methods of drug evaluation.
d. Draw well labelled diagram of TS of fennel fruit. Describe microscopy of fennel fruit.
e. Give chemical constituents and uses of:
   i. Senna   ii. Vinca

Q 3. Attempt any *three* of the following:

a. Describe morphological method of classification of crude drugs along with demerits and merits.
b. Define laxatives. Classify laxatives alongwith examples.
c. Write biological sources and chemical constituents of:
   i. Balsam of tolu   ii. Coriander
d. Describe method of preparation of cotton
e. Which part(s) of following crude drugs is useful as a drug:
   i. Senna   ii. Tulsi
   iii. Vinca   iv. Aconite

Q 4. Attempt any *three* of the following:

a. Describe any two methods of extraction of volatile oil from crude drug.
b. Define diuretics. Write biological source, chief chemical constituents of Punernava.
c. Differentiate between animal fibres and plant fibers.
d. Classify tannins with examples.
e. Give the examples of pharmaceutical aids from animal source and plant source alongwith their uses.

Q 5. Attempt any *three* of the following:

a. Write different types of surgical dressing prepared from cotton and wool.
b. Write biological sources and uses of:
   i. Garlic   ii. Colchicum
   iii. Ginger   iv. Nutmeg
c. Name adulterants and substitutes of:
   i. Senna   ii. Clove

d. Explain morphologic characters of Ipecac or Gokhru with diagram.

e. Define antirheumatics. Explain biological source, chemical constituents and uses of any one drug from this class.

Q 6. Explain chemical tests of following drugs (any *four*):

a. Digitalis	b. Acacia
c. Turmeric	d. Asafoetida
e. Rauwolfia	f. Linseed

Winter Examination 2010
D Pharm First Year
Pharmacognosy

Q 1. Attempt any *ten* of the following:

a. Define pharmacognosy. Who coined the word pharmacognosy?

b. Differentiate between leaf and leaflet.

c. Name the four Traditional Indian Systems of Medicine

d. Define laxatives with two examples.

e. Write two crude drugs for following families:
   i. Leguminosae
   ii. Liliaceae

f. Explain 'Borntrager test' for senna

g. Write about:
   i. Galen   ii. Hippocrates

h. Suggest the crude drug which contain:
   i. Morphine   ii. D-Linalool
   iii. Colchicine   iv. Margosine

i. Which part of plant is used as a drug in case of:
   i. Cinnamon   ii. Clove
   iii. Gokhru   iv. Ephedra

j. Mention two crude drugs for each of the following:
   i. Anti-diabetics   ii. Anti-tussives

k. Define drug evaluation. Enlist physical standard used for evaluation.

l. Mention synonyms of:
   i. Vinca   ii. Nutmeg
   iii. Liquorice   iv. Acacia

Q 2. Attempt any *three* of the following:

a. Differentiate organized and unorganized crude drugs with examples.

b. Describe morphological method of classification of crude drugs with examples.

c. What are volatile oils? Give the general properties of volatile oils.

d. Define drug adulteration. Mention the different methods used for drug adulteration with examples.

e. What are Tannins? Give biological source, chemical constituents and use of (any *one*):

    i. Black catechu   ii. Pale catechu

Q 3. Attempt any *three* of the following:

a. Define and classify resins and resin combinations with examples.

b. Describe the method for preparation of cotton fibre.

c. Explain the general method for isolation of alkaloids.

d. Draw a well labelled diagram of T.S. of ginger and describe the same.

e. What are Alkaloids? Give biological source, chemical constituents and use of (any *one*):

    i. Cinchona   ii. Ipecacuanha

Q 4. Attempt any *three* of the following:

a. Explain the general chemical tests for identification of tannins.

b. What are surgical dressing? Give the ideal requirements of surgical dressings.

c. Describe method of collection of preparation Rauwolfia for market.

d. Write the morphological characters of Umbelliferous fruit along with diagram.

e. What are Vitamins? Give the biological source, chemical constituents and use of (any *one*):

    i. Amla

    ii. Shark liver oil

Q 5. Attempt any *three* of the following:

a. Define and classify sutures with examples.

b. What are Glycosides? Write the tests for cardiac glycosides.

c. Define pharmaceutical aid. Classify according to their use and application with examples.

d. Write the adulterants and substitutes of digitalis.

e. What are enzymes? Give the biological source, chemical constituents and use of (any *one*):

    i. Diastase   ii. Papain

Q 6. Explain chemical tests of the following crude drugs (any *four*):

a. Honey	b. Turmeric
c. Asafoetida	d. Nux vomica
e. Agar	f. Wool

Summer Examination 2011
D Pharm First Year
Pharmacognosy

Q 1. Attempt any *ten* of the following:

a. Who coined the word 'Pharmacognosy' and how?

b. Define antitussives with examples.

c. Define technical products with any four examples.

d. Explain role of "Galen" in the history of pharmacognosy.

e. Which parts of the plant is used as drug?

    i. Pyrethrum   ii. Rauwolfia

    iii. Amla   iv. Digitalis

f. Define and classify tannins with examples

g. Name the drugs which contain:

    i. Colchicine   ii. Emetine

    iii. Vit. A   iv. Mucilage

h. Mention synonyms of following drugs:

    i. Ephedra

    ii. Liquorice

    iii. Nuxvomica

    iv. Honey

i. Name four traditional indigenous systems of medicine in India. What is principle of Ayurveda?

j. Differentiate between Leaf and Leaflet.

k. Write biological source and uses of Guggul.

l. Describe morphological characters of Ginger with diagram.

Q 2. Attempt any *three* of the following:

a. Draw well labelled diagram of TE of fennel and describe the same.

b. Define and classify pharmaceutical aids with examples.

c. Describe method of collection and preparation of senna leaf for market.

d. Name various methods of classification of crude drugs. Give examples of drugs belonging to family—Leguminosae, Umbelliferae.

Q 3. Attempt any *three* of the following:

a. Define surgical dressing. What are ideal requirements of surgical dressings?

b. Define evaluation of crude drugs. Describe moisture content determination or crude fiber.

c. Define resins. How are they classified?

d. Give two examples of drugs belonging to family
  i. Lauraceae   ii. Rutaceae
  iii. Solanaceae   iv. Liliaceae

Q 4. Attempt any *three* of the following:

a. Describe any two terms with examples:
  i. Antidiabetic
  ii. Carminative
  iii. Aphrodiasic
b. What are cardiotonics? Describe biological source and uses of any one cardiotonic drugs.
c. Give biological source, chemical constituents and uses of Vinca.
d. Describe chemical constituents of any *two*:
  i. Black pepper   ii. Nux vomica
  iii. Amla   iv. Liquorice

Q 5. Attempt any *three* of the following:

a. Define and classify alkaloids with examples of crude drugs.
b. Differentiate between organised and unorganized drugs with examples.
c. Define catgut. Differentiate between ligatures and sutures. What are most essential properties of catgut?
d. Differentiate between fixed oil and volatile oil with examples of crude drugs.

Q 6. Explain chemical tests of any *three* crude drugs:

a. Black catachu
b. Shark-liver oil
c. Turmeric
d. Aloe
e. Benzoin

Winter Examination 2011
D Pharm First Year
Pharmacognosy

Q 1. Attempt any *ten* of the following:

a. Define the term carminatives with two examples.
b. Differentiate between Sumatra benzoin and Siam benzoin by giving two chemical tests.

c. Write the properties of alkaloids by giving four points.

d. Define the term pharmaceutical aid. Give the examples of it, obtained from animal source and mineral source.

e. Write the biological source of crude drug from family Flacourtiaceae.

f. Which part of the plant is used as a drug in case of:
   i. Punernava   ii. Aloe
   iii. Myrrh   iv. Ergot

g. Mention synonyms of following crude drug:
   i. Beeswan   ii. Starch
   iii. Amla /   iv. Aconite

h. Write four differentiating points between organized and unorganized crude drugs.

i. Name the drug which contains:
   i. Barbaloin   ii. Pentosan
   iii. Lysergic acid   iv. Quinine

j. Assign the English name of crude drug belonging from the families
   i. Malvaceae   ii. Myrtaceae
   iii. Meliaceae   iv. Myristicaceae

k. Write biological sources with family of:
   i. Cinchona   ii. Tobacco

l. What is Galenical pharmacy? Who discovered it?

Q 2. Attempt any _three_ of the following:

a. Define alkaloids. Write the classification of alkaloids, on the basis of chemical structure present in it, also give one example from each type of alkaloid.

b. Explain various methods of classification of crude drug.

c. Give the chemical constituents and uses of:
   i. Gokhru
   ii. Gymnema

d. Explain different means of adulteration of crude drug with suitable examples.

e. Define the term resin. Write about the various combinations of resins.

Q 3. Attempt any _three_ of the following:

a. Write minimum eight characteristics of umbelliferous fruits.

b. Explain the term alternative system of medicine. Explain in detail Ayurvedic system of medicine.

c. Draw a well labelled diagram of T.S. of Senna leaf.

d. Define the term substituents and adulterants. Write the same for the crude drugs clove.

e. Write biological source, family, chemical constituents and uses of 'Ajwain'.

Q 4. Attempt any _three_ of the following:

    a. Define the term fiber. Assign the name of fibre, which is obtained from animal source. Write the biological source and uses of it.

    b. Write minimum eight differentiating pints between volatile oil and fixed oil.

    c. Write short note on 'hemp'.

    d. Explain minimum four chemical tests for turmeric.

    e. Write the biological source of opium, alongwith collection and preparation of it for market.

Q 5. Attempt any _three_ of the following:

    a. Draw a well labelled diagram of T.S. of crude drug, which is used as an antidysenterics.

    b. Explain the life cycle of ergot with diagram.

    c. Give chemical constituents and uses of 'Caster oil'.

    d. Describe the method of preparation of silk from silk cocoons.

    e. Define the term antirheumatics and diuretics with two examples from each category.

Q 6. Explain chemical tests of following crude drugs (any _four_):

    a. Senna

    b. Digitalis

    c. Datura

    d. Nux vomica

    e. Asafoetida

    f. Honey

Summer Examination 2012
D Pharm First Year
Pharmacognosy

Q 1. Answer any _ten_ of the following:

    a. Define pharmacognosy. Who coined the word pharmacognosy?

    b. Write about:

        i. Hippocrates

        ii. Galen

    c. Differentiate: Organised and unorganised crude drugs.

    d. Which part of plant is used as a drug in case of:

        i. Aloe

        ii. Senna

        iii. Rauwolfia

        iv. Cardamom

e. Define 'Diuretics' with two examples.

f. Name the drugs having following synonyms:
    i. Periwinkle   ii. Banda soap
    iii. Ma-huang   iv. Monkshood

g. Explain borntragger test of senna.

h. Name two examples of each of the following:
    i. Antitussives   ii. Antidiabetics

i. Mention the family of following crude drugs:
    i. Colchicum   ii. Tragacanth
    iii. Vasaka   iv. Ashwagandha

j. Suggest the drug contain following chemical constituents:
    i. Margosine   ii. Pentosan
    iii. Bassorin   iv. Reserpine

k. What are natural pesticides? Give two examples.

l. Write the pharmacological action of:
    i. Opium
    ii. Ipecac
    iii. Arjuna
    iv. Castor oil

Q 2. Answer any *three* of the following:

a. Describe morphological method of classification of crude drugs with merits and demerits.

b. What are Cardiotonics? Write adulterants and substitutes of Digitalis.

c. Define 'Resins and Resin combinations'. Classify it with suitable examples.

d. Draw a well labelled diagram of T.S. of Clove or cinchona and describe it.

e. Give the name of the drug which passes the following test and explain it:
    i. Vitali—Morin test
    ii. Swelling factor test

Q 3. Answer any *three* of the following:

a. Define 'Drug evaluation'. Explain 'organoleptic' method for evaluation of crude drugs.

b. Describe external characters of fennel with diagrams.

c. What are alkaloids? Explain, how the alkaloids are extracted from plant?

d. Describe the method of preparation of cotton fibres.

e. Explain:
    i. Stomatal no.   ii. Vein Islet no with example

Q 4. Answer any *three* of the following:

a. What are vitamins? Write the biological source, chemical constituents and uses of shark liver oil or Amla.

b. Describe method of cultivation, collection and preparation of rauwolfia.

c. What are volatile oils? Give the general properties of volatile oils.

d. Define sutures and ligatures. Write the ideal requirements of sutures.

e. Name the drug and their uses belongs to following family (any *two*):
  i. Myristicaceae   ii. Burseraceae
  iii. Lauraceae.

Q 5. Answer any *three* of the following:

a. Define 'Drug adulteration'. Describe any three methods of adulteration with suitable examples.

b. Write biological source, chemical constituents and uses of ergot.

c. What are tannins? Write the general chemical tests of tannins.

d. Define 'pharmaceutical aids'. Classify according to their sources.

e. Describe any *two* terms with examples:
  i. Disinfectant   ii. Purgative
  iii. Carminatives.

Q 6. Explain chemical tests of following crude drugs (any *four*):

a. Clove   b. Acacia
c. Turmeric   d. Wool
e. Nux vomica   f. Gelatin

Winter Examination 2012
D Pharm First Year
Pharmacognosy

Q 1. Answer any *eight* of the following:

a. Define:
  i. Pharmacognosy   ii. Crude drugs

b. Which parts of the plant is used as a drug in case of:
  i. Punarnava   ii. Ephedra
  iii. Nutmeg   iv. Arjuna

c. Name the drug which contains the following constituents:
  i. Rhein   ii. Vit. C
  iii. Fenchone   iv. Bassorin

d. Mention synonyms of the following drugs:
  i. Tulsi   ii. Nux vomica
  iii. Pyrethrum   iv. Cinchona

   e. Explain in brief principles of Ayurveda.

   f. Differentiate between gums and resins.

   g. Define 'Astringents'. Give any two examples.

   h. Explain why Borntrager's test is modified for Aloes?

   i. Explain the contribution of Galen in the development of pharmacognosy.

   j. Write biological source and uses of vinca.

   k. Name the family of following drugs:

      i. Rauwolfia

      ii. Clove

      iii. Gokhru

      iv. Guggul

   l. Draw well labelled diagram showing external morphological characters of nux vomica.

Q 2. Answer any *four* of the following:

   a. Explain pharmacological method of classification with its advantages and disadvantages.

   b. Define 'alkaloids'. Explain any two tests for their identification.

   d. Describe external characters of Umbelliferous fruits. Give any two examples.

   e. What are the official requirements of surgical dressing?

   f. What are 'Terpenoids'? Classify them.

Q 3. Answer any *four* of the following:

   a. Describe organoleptic method of evaluation.

   b. Differentiate between antiseptics and disinfections.

   c. What are balsams? Name any two balsamic drugs.

   d. Give biological source and uses of digitalis.

   e. Give any three general tests for identification of tannins.

   f. Classify glycosides on the basis of linkage between sugar and non-sugar with one example from each.

Q 4. Answer any *four* of the following:

   a. Draw well labelled diagram of T.S. of nux vomical or clove.

   b. Give biological source, chemical constituents and uses of Vasaka.

   c. What is 'Garbling'? How senna is collected and prepared for market?

   d. What are bulk laxatives? Give biological source of any one drug use as bulk laxative.

   e. Explain with suitable example how stomatal no. helps in evaluation of leaf drugs.

   f. Differentiate between plant fibre and animal fibre.

Q 5. Answer any *four* of the following:

a. Define 'Drug adulteration'. Explain any four method of drug adulteration with examples.

b. What are pharmaceutical aids? Give any four classes with example.

c. Differentiate between volatile oils and fixed oils.

d. Enlist the parameters under physical evaluation.

e. Give biological source of absorbent cotton. How is it prepared?

f. Define 'Oxytocics'. Name chemical constituents of drug used as oxytocics.

Q 6. Explain chemical tests of following (any *four*):

a. Clove   b. Shark-liver oil

c. Senna   d. Asafoetida

e. Turmeric   f. Gelatin

Summer Examination 2013
D Pharm First Year
Pharmacognosy

Q 1. Attempt any *ten* of the following:

a. Define pharmacognosy. Who wrote the book 'Analecta pharmacognostica'?

b. Explain the role of 'Galen' in the history of pharmacognosy.

c. What are balsams? Name the balsams used in pharmacy.

d. Define with examples:
    i. Antitussives   ii. Diuretics

e. Which part of the plant is used as drug?
    i. Gymnema   ii. Clove
    iii. Black pepper   iv. Rauwolfia

f. Mention the synonyms of following:
    i. Pyrethrum   ii. Nutmeg
    iii. Cinnamon   iv. Ephedra

g. Name the drug having following family:
    i. Rubiaceae   ii. Burseraceae
    iii. Zingiberaceae   iv. Euphorbiaceae

h. Write biological source, with family:
    i. Honey   ii. Shatavari

i. Write the morphological characters of fennel with diagram.

j. Name the drug which contain
    i. Aconitine   ii. Colchicine
    iii. Emetine   iv. Vit. A

k. Explain 'gold beater skin test' for tannins.

l. Name the four drugs acting on nervous system.

Q 2. Attempt any *three* of the following:

a. Write the merits and demerits of morphological method of classification.

b. Define drug adulteration. Explain any two methods of drug adulteration with examples.

c. Draw a well labelled T.S. diagram of nux vomical and describe the dame by giving four points.

d. Define volatile oil. Classify with examples.

e. What are Glycosides? Give the biological source, chemical constituents and uses of any one.

    i. Digitalis   ii. Senna

Q 3. Attempt any *three* of the following:

a. Define drug evaluation. Explain, whey moisture content is important for drug evaluation?

b. Describe the general method for extraction of alkaloids.

c. Differentiate between organized and unorganized crude drugs by giving four points.

d. What are surgical dressings? Give the ideal requirements of surgical dressings.

e. Define Tannins. Give the biological source, chemical constituents and uses of any one.

    i. Black catechu   ii. Pale catechu

Q 4. Attempt any *three* of the following:

a. Define and classify resins and resin combinations with examples.

b. Describe the method of preparation of cotton or silk fibres.

c. Differentiate between volatile oils and fixed oils by giving eight points.

d. Explain the term enzymes with its general properties. Write biological source and uses of enzyme papain.

e. Define perfumes and flavouring agents. Give the biological source, chemical constituents of any one.

    i. Sandalwood   ii. Mentha oil.

Q 5. Attempt any *three* of the following:

a. What are terpenoids? Give general properties of terpenoids by giving six points.

b. Define and classify pharmaceutical aids with examples.

c. Describe the cultivation, collection and preparation of opium for market.

d. Define sutures and ligatures. Give the official ideal requirements of surgical dressings.

e. Explain life cycle of ergot with diagram

Q 6. Explain minimum *three* chemical tests for each of the following (any *four*):

a. Acacia
b. Turmeric
c. Asafoetida
d. Rhubarb
e. Wool
f. Gelatin

Winter Examination 2013
D Pharm First Year
Pharmacognosy

Q 1. Attempt any *ten*:

a. Write family of:
  i. Tulsi
  ii. Neem
  iii. Cinchona
  iv. Aconite

b. Write name of drug which contains:
  i. Eugenol
  ii. Basorin
  iii. Fenchone
  iv. Codeine.

c. Write name of drug for which following chemical test is applied:
  i. Keller Killiani test
  ii. Borntrager test
  iii. Klunge's test
  iv. Halphene's test

d. Write name of drug which have following synonym:
  i. Nux moschata
  ii. Foxglove leaves
  iii. Cera flava
  iv. Indian saffron

e. Which name of drug used as:
  i. Carminative
  ii. Expectorant
  iii. Antiseptic
  iv. Diuretic

f. Define and write one example of:
  i. Astringents
  ii. Purgative

g. Which part of plant is used as drug in case of:
  i. Clove
  ii. Ginger
  iii. Pyrethrum
  iv. Tobacco

h. Define 'Crude drug'. Write the contribution of 'galen' in the development of pharmacognosy.

i. What is vitamin? Write names of drugs which contain vitamin A and vitamin C.

j. Write the morphological characters of 'Fennel' with diagram.

k. Write about Charak and Seydler.

l. Write chemical constituents and uses of ergot.

Q 2. Attempt any *three*:

   a. Draw well labelled diagram of T.S. of cinchona and describe, its microscopy by giving four points.

   b. Define and classify alkaloids, according to basic chemical structure.

   c. Define drug evaluation. Describe microscopic method.

   d. Describe method of collection and preparation of digitalis for market.

   e. Write biological source, chemical constituents and uses of Rauwolfia.

Q 3. Attempt any *three*:

   a. Describe chemical method of classification of crude drug with its merits and demerits.

   b. Define adulteration. Write methods of adulteration with example.

   c. What are lipids? Define fixed oil. Write its properties and uses.

   d. Differentiate between:

      i. Gum and mucillage

      ii. Organised and unorganised crude drugs.

   e. What is ash value? Write its type and importance in evaluation of drugs.

Q 4. Attempt any *three*:

   a. Write biological source, chemical constituents and uses of cinnamon.

   b. Describe method of preparation of surgical cotton.

   c. Define and classify pharmaceutical aids with example.

   e. Define resin. Write about resin combinations with example.

Q 5. Attempt any *three*:

   a. Define the term 'Antileprotic'. Write the name, biological source and chemical constituents of it.

   b. Name the drug from family Burseraceae, along with its chemical constituents and uses.

   c. Define sutures and write ideal requirements of sutures.

   d. Describe different shapes of barks with diagrams.

   e. Define volatile oils. Explain methods of extraction of volatile oil.

Q 6. Write chemical tests of crude drugs (any *four*):

   a. Black catechu

   b. Starch

   c. Agar

   d. Benzoin

   e. Asatoetida

   f. Nux vomica

Winter Examination 2014
D Pharm First Year
Pharmacognosy

Q 1. Attempt any *ten* of the following:

a. Define the term "Antiseptics' and 'Disinfectants'.

b. Define the term cardiotonics. Give the biological source with family of any one cardiotonic drug.

c. Which part of the plant is used as a drug in case of:
  i. Ergot
  ii. Rauwolfia
  iii. Black catechu
  iv. Indian bdellium

d. Mention synonym of following crude drug:
  i. Bees wax
  ii. Ephedra
  iii. Datura
  iv. Turmeric

e. Mention two examples of drug for which each of the following part are used
  i. Dried juice
  ii. Dried aqueous extract

f. Write the minimum four characteristics features of umbelliferous fruits.

g. Write four differentiating points between organised and unorganised crude drug.

h. Name the drug which contains following active chemical constituents:
  i. Lysergic acid
  ii. Asaresinolannol
  iii. Brucine
  iv. Reserpine

i. Name the one drug which belongs to following family:
  i. Rutaceae   ii. Burscraceae
  iii. Apidae   iv. Lauraceae

j. Which chemical substance is responsible for pungent taste of:
  i. Ginger   ii. Ajwain

k. Describe the contribution of following persons in development in pharmacognosy
  i. Hippocrates
  ii. Galen

l. Write two chemical tests for identification of nux vomica

Q 2. Attempt any *three* of the following:

    a. Explain the life cycle of Ergot with diagram.

    b. Describe the method of preparation of cotton fibres.

    c. Name the drug which is used as antimalarial. Write biological source with family and chemical constituents on it.

    d. Define adulteration and substitution. Write the adulterants of:

        i. Clove

        ii. Digitalis

Q 3. Attempt any *three* of the following:

    a. Define 'Resin'. Give the name, synonyms and biological source of drug which contain Δ' THC in it.

    b. Give minimum two differentiating chemical tests in between:

        i. Summatra benzoin and siam benzoin

        ii. Black catechu and Pale catechu

    c. Explain different means of adulteration of crude drug with suitable examples.

    d. Draw well labeled diagram of T.S of 'Clove' along with its microscopy by giving four points.

Q 4. Attempt any *three* of the following:

    a. Explain in detail the scope of Pharmacognosy.

    b. What are alkaloids? Explain how the alkaloids are extracted from plant.

    c. What do you mean by 'Swelling factor'? Describe how will you determine it? According to I.P what should be the swelling factor of Isabgol?

    d. Write biological source with family, chemical constituents and uses of 'Opium'.

Q 5. Attempt any *three* of the following:

    a. Write minimum eight differentiating points between volatile oil and fixed oil.

    b. Write biological source with family of Rauwolfia. Describe method of collection and preparation of Rauwolfia for market.

    c. Define the term Diuretics and carminatives with two examples from each category.

    d. Write the detail methods of isolation of volatile oils.

Q 6. Explain chemical tests of following crude drugs (any *four*):

    a. Starch   b. Shark liver oil

    c. Turmeric   d. Datura

    e. Acacia   f. Digitalis

Summer Examination 2015
D Pharm First Year
Pharmacognosy

Q 1. Attempt any *ten* of the following:

    a. Define pharmacognosy. Give the contribution of Hippocrates.

    b. Name a drug having following microscopical characters:

        i. Lignified trichomes

        ii. Paracytic stomata

    c. Differentiate between organised crude drug and unorganised crude drug.

    d. Mention the synonym of the following drugs:

        i. Asafoetida   ii. Gymnema

        iii. Chaulmoogra oil   iv. Dioscorea

    e. Write down the biological source of the following drugs:

        i. Cinchona

        ii. Vinca

    f. Draw a well-labelled diagram showing morphological characters of 'Coriander fruit'.

    g. Give the example of a drug used as antihypertensive and write its biological source.

    h. Identify a drug containing following chemical constituents:

        i. Bassorin   ii. Kinoin

        iii. Margosine   iv. Fibroin

    i. Enlist various Indian traditional system of medicine.

    j. Give any two examples of drugs from Umbelliferae family and mention two characteristic features of umbelliferous fruits.

    k. Define oxytocics. Write down chemical constituents of ergot.

    l. Give the examples of drugs from the following families:

        i. Rubiaceae   ii. Polygonaceae

        iii. Acantheaceae   iv. Rutaceae

Q 2. Answer any *three* of the following:

    a. Explain pharmacological method of classification of crude drug with its merits and demerits.

    b. Mention the adulterants and substituents of:

        i. Clove

        ii. Senna

    c. Define natural pesticide. Give the biological source, chemical constituents, and uses of any one drug.

    d. Define lipids. Write down the properties of fixed oil.

    e. Differentiate between plant fibre and animal fibre.

Q 3. Attempt any _three_ of the following:

  a. Give the uses of:

      i. Rauwolfia   ii. Ispaghula

      iii. Colchicum   iv. Garlic

  b. Draw a well-labelled diagram of T.S. of ginger and describe it.

  c. Define tannins and write down the chemical test for identification of tannins.

  d. Describe any four physical methods of evaluation of crude drug.

  e. Define suture and ligature and write down the properties of it.

Q 4. Attempt any _three_ of the following:

  a. Write down the classification of Glycosides on the basis of linkage between sugar and non-sugar with one example each.

  b. Name a drug containing papain and citral as active constituents and write their uses.

  c. Define Diuretic. Give the examples of it and write biological source, chemical constituents of any one drug.

  d. How will you differentiate black catechu and pale catechu?

  e. Give the method of collection and preparation of opium for market.

Q 5. Attempt any _three_ of the following:

  a. Define pharmaceutical aids. Give the classification of it with examples.

  b. Give the biological source and chemical constituents of:

      i. Amla   ii. Sandalwood

  c. Define drug evaluation and explain the terms:

      i. Stomatal No.   ii. Stomatal index

      iii. Vein-islet No.

  d. Define:

      i. Antidysenteric

      ii. Enzymes

      iii. Vitamins

      iv. Antileprotics

  e. Describe the method of preparation of silk fibres.

Q 6. Explain the chemical tests for following crude drugs (any _four_):

  a. Starch

  b. Myrrh

  c. Tolu balsam

  d. Digitalis

  e. Asafoetida

  f. Gelatin

Winter Examination 2015
D Pharm First Year
Pharmacognosy

Q 1. Attempt any *ten* of the following:

a. Define crude drug. Write two examples of crude drugs obtained from natural source.

b. What are enzymes? Write two examples.

c. Name the two crude drugs which are used as:
   i. Coloring agent   ii. Sweetening agent

d. Who is described as "FATHER OF MEDICINE"? Why?

e. Which part of the plant is used as crude drugs in case of the following?
   i. Black pepper
   ii. Ajowan
   iii. Picrorrhiza
   iv. Dioscorea

f. Why saponin glycosides are not safe for intravenous administration? Explain.

g. Which drug is found to contain?
   i. Ferulic acid
   ii. Hydrocarpic acid
   iii. Vascicinone
   iv. Ascorbic acid

h. Name the drugs having following synonym.
   i. Puncture vine
   ii. Crow fig
   iii. Insect flower
   iv. Marihuana

i. What is Ayurveda? Describe contribution of "Sushrut".

j. Differentiate between organised and unorganised drugs.

k. Write biological source and uses of lemon grass oil.

1. Describe morphological characters of hyocyamus with diagram.

Q 2. Attempt any *three* of the following:

a. Draw well labelled diagram of transverse section of Nux Vomica and describe the same.

b. What is evaluation of crude drug? Describe Ash value as a criteria in evaluation.

c. Mention six methods of classification of crude drugs. Write advantages and disadvantages of taxonomical method of classification.

d. What are barks? Describe three methods of collection at barks.

Q 3. Attempt any *three* of the following:

a. What are balsams? Give one chemical test for identification of cinnamic acid. Write its biological source.
b. What are sutures ? Write ideal properties of sutures.
c. Define each of the following with example.
  i. Antiseptic
  ii. Substitute
  iii. Carminative
  iv. Astringent
d. Name two drugs containing following chemical group or structure.
  i. Tropaine alkaloid
  ii. True tannins
  iii. Cyanogenetic glycosides
  iv. Natural wax

Q 4. Attempt any *three* of the following:

a. Define the following with examples (any **two**):
  i. Oxytocic
  ii. Anthelmintic
  iii. Galactogogue
b. What are vitamins? Describe biological source, chemical constituents and uses of any one crude drug containing vitamin.
c. Describe life cycle of ergot.
d. Give biological source and chemical constituents of following drugs:
  i. Digitalis
  ii. Aloes
  iii. Cinnamon
  iv. Ephedra

Q 5. Attempt any *three* of the following:

a. Describe important characteristic of four adulterants of 'Clove.'
b. What is nutmeg mace? Describe chemical constituents and uses of it.
c. As a technical product write uses of gelatin and pectin.
d. Differentiate between raw cotton and surgical cotton.

Q 6. Explain any *two* chemical tests each of any *three* of the following crude drugs:

a. Myrrh
b. Honey
c. Gelatin
d. Castor oil

Summer Examination 2016
D Pharm First Year
Pharmacognosy

Q 1. Answer any *eight* of the following:

a. Define pharmacognosy. When and who coined the term pharmacognosy?

b. Name the drug which contains:
   i. Bassorin
   ii. Harmine
   iii. Fenchone
   iv. Reserpine

c. Mention a crude drug for which each of the following synonym is applicable:
   i. Mel
   ii. Oleum selachoids
   iv. Yam
   v. Cera flava

d. Name a crude drug to which each of the following chemical test is applicable:
   i. Klunge's test
   ii. Fiche's test
   iii. Vitali-Morin test
   iv. Keller-Killiani test

e. Mention which part of the plant is useful as a drug in case of:
   i. Gymnema
   ii. Nutmeg
   iii. Liquorice
   iv. Black pepper

f. For identification of which crude drugs swelling factor is determined. Describe how will you determine it.

g. Write chemical tests for ergot.

h. Describe method of preparation of cotton.

i. What are balsams? Name balsams used in pharmacy.

j. What do you know about 'Ayurveda' as traditional Indian system of medicines?

Q 2. Answer any *four* of the following:

a. Give two examples of crude drugs from family:
   i. Burseraceae
   ii. Apocyanaceae
   iii. Scrophulariaceae

b. Define evaluation of crude drugs. Describe any two microscopical methods of drug evaluation.

c. What are surgical dressings? Give the ideal requirements of surgical dressings.

d. Define and classify pharmaceutical aids with examples.

e. Differentiate between organised and unorganised crude drugs with examples.

    f. Define perfumes and flavouring agents. Give biological source and chemical constituents of any one:
   - i. Peppermint oil
   - ii. Lemon grass oil

Q 3. Answer any *four* of the following:
   - a. Define volatile oil. Explain method of isolation of volatile oil.
   - b. (i) What are enzymes? Give biological source of diastase.
     (ii) Define tannins. Write chemical test for tannins.
   - c. Describe pharmacological method of classification with its merits and demerits.
   - d. Draw a well-labelled cellular diagram of T.S. of bark used as antimalarial. Describe any two microscopic characters.
   - e. Describe method of collection and preparation of digitalis for market.
   - f. Write biological source, chemical constituents and uses of garlic.

Q 4. Answer any *four* of the following:
   - a. How will you differentiate:
     - i. Plant fibres and animal fibres
     - ii. Leaf and leaflet
   - b. Define antiseptic. Give biological source, chemical constituents of benzoin.
   - c. Write biological source and use of:
     - i. Neem   ii. Shatavari
   - d. Define sutures and ligatures. Write ideal requirements of sutures.
   - e. Explain the significance of following in evaluation of crude drugs with suitable examples:
     - i. Alcohol soluble extractives
     - ii. Optical rotation
   - f. Define resin and resin combinations. Classify it with suitable examples.

Q 5. Answer any *four* of the following:
   - a. Define and classify alkaloids with examples of crude drugs.
   - b. Write the morphological characters of ipecac along with diagram.
   - c. Define adulteration. Give various methods of adulteration with suitable examples.
   - d. Which umbelliferous fruit mainly contains a chemical constituent linalol? Write its morphological characters with diagram.
   - e. Define with examples of crude drugs (any **three**):
     - i. Oxytocics
     - ii. Astringents

    iii. Carminatives

    iv. Antitumour

  f. Define diuretics. Write biological source, chemical constituents of punarnava.

Q 6. Write chemical tests of crude drugs (any *four*):

  a. Nux vomica   b. Turmeric

  c. Shark liver oil   d. Datura

  e. Wool   f. Acacia

Winter Examination 2016
D Pharm First Year
Pharmacognosy

Q 1. Attempt any *eight* of the following:

  a. Define with example (any **two**):

    i. Dried juices

    ii. Latex

    iii. Extracts

  b. Differentiate between Leaf and Leaflets.

  c. Which part of the plant is used as drug?

    i. Cannabis   ii. Rauwolfia

    iii. Cardamom   iv. Ergot

  d. Explain the role of "Galen" and "Dioscorides" in the development of pharmacognosy.

  e. Name the drug which contains:

    i. Oleo gum resin

    ii. Strychnine, brucine

    iii. Allyl, propyl disulphide, allin, allicinel d-linalool

  f. Describe morphological characters of clove with diagram.

  g. What is the significance of the following chemical tests when wool is treated with:

    i. Lead acetate solution

    ii. Millon's reagent

  h. What are enzymes, give its example.

  i. What is the significance of pharmacopial standards

  j. Write synonyms for each of the following:

    i. Gokhru   ii. Vasaka

    iii. Aconite   iv. Gymnema

  k. Which chemical class is identified by modified Borntrager's test? How will you perform it?

  1. Write official requirement of surgical dressings.

Q 2. Attempt any *Three* of the following:

a   What are volatile oils? State different techniques for isolation of volatile oils.

b. Describe method of collection and preparation of Rauwolfia for market.

c. What are antirheumatics? Describe biological source and uses of any one antirheumatic drug.

d. Describe the synonym, chemical constituent and uses of any two:

   i. Liquorice   ii. Nux Vomica

   iii. Papaya   iv. Tobacco

e. Explain the chemical test for identification of crude drug containing:

   i. Cardiac glycoside

   ii. Tropane alkaloid

Q 3. Attempt any *three* of the following:

a. What are resins? Give the classification of resins.

b. Describe pharmacological method of classification of crude drugs with its advantages and disadvantages.

c. Give any two examples of drugs from each of the following families:

   i. Labiateae   ii. Solanaceae

   iii. Burseraceae   iv. Apocynaceae

d. Explain with diagram, morphological characters of fruit drug belonging to family Umbelliferae.

e. Differentiate between Acacia and Tragacanth.

Q 4. Attempt any *three* of the following:

a. Draw a well-labelled diagram of T.S. of senna describe the same.

b. Describe the method of preparation for cotton fibre.

c. Write about 'Ayurveda' as traditional Indian system of medicines.

d. Write the biological source and uses of:

   i Starch   ii Rhubarb

   iii Neem   iv Wool

e. Define oxytocics. Explain life cycle of ergot.

Q 5. Attempt any *three* of the following:

a. Define adulteration and substitution. Describe why moisture content is useful in evaluation of crude drug.

b. Give the classification of alkaloids with one example of each type and their source.

c. How will you differentiate:

   i. Organised and unorganised crude drugs.

   ii. Siam benzoin and Sumatra benzoin.

    d. Name the drug used as Antimalarial. Give its synonym, biological source and chemical constituent.

    e. Define with two examples:

       i. Carminatives

       ii. Astringents

Q 6. Explain the chemical tests of any *four* crude drugs:

    a. Myrrh

    b. Shark liver oil

    c. Turmeric

    d. Gelatin

    e. Asafoetida

    f. Black catechu

Summer Examination 2017
D Pharm First Year
Pharmacognosy

Q 1. Attempt any *ten* of the following:

    a. Define antitussive and antiseptics.

    b. What is Galenical pharmacy and who is called as 'Father of Medicine'?

    c. Name the drug which contains:

       i. Glycyrrhizin   ii. Amylase

       iii. D-linalool   iv. Quinine

    d. Differentiate between Roots and Rhizomes.

    e. Describe morphological characters of Nux Vomica seed with diagram.

    f. What is the significance of 'Modified Borntrager test'? Explain how it is performed.

    g. Mention synonyms of the following drugs:

       i. Nutmeg   ii. Rauwolfia

       iii. Vasaka   iv. Linseed

    h. Define:

       i. Palisade ratio   ii. Stomatal index

    i. What are the official requirements of surgical dressings?

    j. Which part of the plant is used as drug in case of:

       i. Picrorrhiza   ii. Amla

       iii. Belladonna   iv. Colchicum

    k. Write the biological source of:

       i. Gymnema   ii. Gokhru

    l. Write any two therapeutic uses of tannins with suitable examples.

Q 2. Attempt any *three* of the following:

    a. What are umbelliferous fruits? Describe morphological characters of umbelliferous fruits with diagram.

    b. Define enzymes. Write biological source, chemical constituents and uses of Papaya.

    c. How will you distinguish silk fibre from wool fibres?

    d. Describe chemical method of classification of crude drug with its merits and demerits.

    e. i. Mention the adulterants of honey and explain the chemical test for detection of adulterants.

       ii. Enlist the four species of cinchona.

Q 3. Attempt any *three* of the following:

    a. Describe method of preparation of silk fibre. Give biological source of silk.

    b. i. Give biological source and uses of drug which contain 'Bassorin' as a chemical constituents.

       ii. What are natural pesticides : Give two examples.

    c. Draw a well-labelled diagram of T.S. of ipecac and describe it.

    d. Define laxatives. Write the biological source, chemical constituents of leaf which has laxative action.

    e. Define 'Resins and Resin combinations'. Classify it with suitable examples.

Q 4. Attempt any *three* of the following:

    a. Write the synonyms, chemical constituents and uses of dried Kernel of family Myristicaceae.

    b. Explain the significance of following in evaluation of crude drug with suitable examples:

       i. Optical rotation

       ii. Moisture content

    c. Describe the method of cultivation and collection of opium for market.

    d. Define glycosides. Describe the method for extraction of glycosides.

    e. i. What is garbling?

       ii. Write about contribution of Seydler.

Q 5. Attempt any *three* of the following;

    a. Give chemical constituents and uses of following: (any **two**)

       i. Vinca

       ii. Tolu balsam

       iii. Chaulmoogra oil

       iv. Neem

    b. Define and classify pharmaceutical aids with examples.

    c. Define cardiotonics. Give the biological source and chemical constituents of any one drug.

    d. Write the adulterants and substitute for:
       i. Acacia
      ii. Nux Vomica

    e. How is quantitative microscopical evaluation done? Explain it.

Q 6. Explain chemical tests for following crude drug (any *four*):

    a. Black catechu

    b. Myrrh

    c. Ergot

    d. Kaolin

    e. Agar

    f. Shark liver oil